ASIANS I

Caring for Hindus and their Families:
religious aspects of care

Alix Henley

C

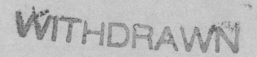

HEC/DHSS/King Edward's Hospital Fund for London

Acknowledgements

I should like to thank all the people who have helped me put this book together and who have given so much of their time and energy to the task. In particular I should like to thank Sushil Daru, Lopa Daru, Catherine Ballard, Roger Ballard, Rupert Snell, Meena Bhatia, Shakuntala Dadhwal, Ashok Basudev, Mira Manek, Ros Morpeth, Pandit Vishnu Narayan, Balmukund Parikh, Nina Patel, Praful Patel, and Banu Vaghela. Their contributions have been invaluable and their patience extraordinary.

I hope there is nothing in the book that offends them, though I am sure there is a good deal that they would consider could be improved or refined. I apologise for any errors or infelicities and take full responsibility for them. They and other readers will understand how difficult it is to compress such a subject into a small book; on the other hand I take comfort in knowing that Hinduism in its vastness and complexity will survive my small attempts completely unruffled.

I should also like to thank Dreen Daniels for her patient typing and re-typing, Fred and my family for their love and support, and Graham Cannon at the King's Fund and Ted Gang at the Department of Health for supporting and encouraging me through this project.

Translations from the Bhagavad Gita are taken from *The Bhagavad Gita* trans. Juan Mascaro (Penguin Classics 1975) pp. 50, 74–5, 82, 101, 102, and 119, copyright © Juan Mascaro 1962, and are reprinted by permission of Penguin Books Ltd.

Alix Henley
June 1983

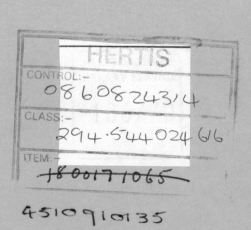

Contents

Table

Maps

Like a member of any other religion, a Hindu is many things at different times and places. However, there is some form of a basic unity in this diversity, and the Hindu has a rich heritage: a universe created by a Superconsciousness, a Supreme Being, which also resides in his or her inner self; a precise configuration of stars and planets existing at the time of birth, which shapes his or her destiny; a legacy of ancient and ageless philosophy of life, initially revealed but later enshrined in crisp and terse poetic stanzas pregnant with deep meaning; an intuitive view of life that serves as a sheet anchor through moments of joy and pain; a continuum of good and evil in thought and deed which the Hindu carries from one birth to another, a plethora of gods and saints, idols and images, do's and don'ts, reason and miracles, work and worship, foods and festivals, customs and ceremonies in life, birth and death.

Sushil Daru
November 1982

1. General introduction

Ideas, beliefs and practices based on religion are central to the lives of many Asian people in Britain. They tend to become even more important at times of personal crisis and isolation such as during illness and in hospital, when people are also most likely to be dependent on the caring services.

An informed understanding of the religious beliefs and values of individual patients is clearly essential to good patient care. No health worker would consciously refuse a patient's request that was connected with his or her religious beliefs or practices. But where health workers do not know very much about a patient's religion they may easily give unintentional offence, especially in the press of daily business.

For example, health workers in Britain usually know the significance of prayer books and crucifixes, and how to avoid causing unnecessary offence when preparing Christian patients for surgery. They are likely to be less confident when a Muslim child comes into hospital with a cloth pouch attached to his arm, or a Sikh patient protests when being shaved for an operation.

The way in which British institutions organise health care has also grown up to fit in with the traditional ways of British society, which are largely based on Christian practices; for example, we try to send patients home over Christmas, Christian chaplains make regular rounds of hospital wards, and Christian services are held on hospital premises. When patients in hospital wish to make confession, to receive communion, or to baptise their babies, ward staff generally understand what to do, and, equally important, are immediately sympathetic to requests. Non-Christian patients often find it more difficult to get help in fulfilling their religious duties merely because these duties are unfamiliar to staff. This increases patients' feelings of unhappiness and

1

isolation.

Few British health workers, or other professionals in the caring services, have up to now been given the opportunity to understand much about the beliefs and practices of Hindus, Sikhs and Muslims. This may inhibit their ability to offer comfort to Asian patients and their families. It may also mean that when patients request special facilities, or refuse to do something for religious reasons, they are regarded with suspicion or irritation.

Asian people in Britain

Most people from the Indian subcontinent and East Africa now living in Britain came from societies in which ideas, values and practices based on religion are taken for granted. Religious events are often the main social events, and religious observances are a normal part of day-to-day individual and community life. Social, philosophical and religious values are intertwined and people may not distinguish them: most acts have religious significance, and a person judges them accordingly.

The extent to which individuals in Britain maintain their religion varies a good deal:

In the early days of settlement, most people felt under great pressure to conform, and to become as inconspicuous as possible in an alien society. This often led them to abandon external religious practices and observances. For example, many Sikh men cut their hair and removed their turbans, because it was believed that this would make it easier for them to get jobs. Some orthodox Hindus began to eat non-vegetarian food to fit in with the British way of life.

As the wives and children of the early Asian settlers began to arrive in Britain, the quality of life within their communities started to improve. The different communities organised places in which to gather and worship. They began to employ permanent religious functionaries to lead prayers and to perform ceremonies that had previously been neglected. As communities grew more established and organised, it became easier for people to practise their religion and to feel supported in their beliefs. Evening or weekend schools were set up, where children could be taught the basic elements of their parents' faith and learn to

2

read the holy books.

This movement was strengthened with the arrival of Asian people from East Africa, who had already had the experience of recreating their way of life and religious identities in a foreign country. They were often familiar, for example, with the practical details of administering temple, gurdwara and mosque committees, and of organising religious ceremonies and festivals within a wider society that did not share their beliefs. In some cases, people from East Africa took over the administration and organisation of Asian religious facilities in Britain.

Diversity and change

There is naturally a great diversity of religious belief and practice among Hindus, Sikhs and Muslims in Britain, just as there is among British Christians. Some people find the focus of their lives in their religion and are extremely devout; others have discarded most external signs and practices but may retain the values of the religion in which they were brought up.

Among young Hindus, Sikhs and Muslims growing up in Britain there is as much diversity of religious belief and practice as there is among their Christian peers. However, their education in British schools and in a Christian-based society with a strong secular emphasis is unlikely to have helped them towards any knowledge or understanding of their parents' beliefs. Some young Asians may also have picked up the racist and negative attitudes towards their cultures that exist among the majority community. This may affect their view of their parents' religion and origins. The degree of young people's understanding and faith will therefore depend largely on their parents and on the provision made by their own communities. Some young Hindus, Sikhs and Muslims are well informed about their faith and are very devout. Others who are not may nevertheless wish to retain some religious practices, particularly when they are ill or in hospital.

This book

This book concentrates on those features of Hindu religious practice that are likely to be particularly important for health workers and other professionals in hospital and in the community, setting them in the context of Hindu religious beliefs and values. It also suggests areas where Hindu practice and custom may conflict with established Health Service provision. It is likely to be especially, but not only, relevant to those Hindus who arrived in Britain as adults.

The material should provide professional workers with a basis of knowledge from which to discuss with practising Hindus their needs and wishes in an informed and sensitive way, bearing in mind that most Hindus are very happy to talk about their beliefs and way of life with sympathetic enquirers.

2. What is Hinduism?

Hinduism is the religion of most of the people of India (over 80 per cent of the total population of about 638 million). It is however much more than what most Western people would think of as a religion. It is a social system and a way of life, as well as a set of beliefs, values and religious practices, and a way of understanding the world. Hinduism can almost be defined as the whole way of life of the majority of Indian people. Hindu religious, philosophical and social values cannot be separated; a Hindu who obeys the social codes and customs laid down for him or her is also fulfilling a religious duty.

It may perhaps be easier to understand Hinduism if one begins by contrasting it with those religions with which most people in Britain are more familiar, Christianity and Judaism, and also with Islam.

Hinduism has evolved in India over four or five thousand years and has been influenced by several incoming cultures and civilisations. Unlike Christianity or Islam, Hinduism has no single founder or major prophet from whom all events are dated; no one person whose words and actions are taken as a source of guidance. It has no single holy book to which all believers refer. It has been, and continues to be, shaped by many different developments of thought and practice, and by several holy scriptures. It is an amalgam of many religious traditions, both national and local.

Hinduism has no church; that is, no central decision-making organisation to prescribe religious dogmas or uniform rules for all its followers; it has no authoritative body to reject certain beliefs or practices as heretical and non-Hindu. There is no central hierarchy of spiritual leaders to control and define Hinduism, or to hand down one universally accepted set of beliefs or practices from generation to generation. Hindus recognise that there are many ways in which an individual may follow his or her religion, and that all lead ultimately to the same goal.

Consequently, it is difficult to specify the exact ways in which individuals will worship, the customs they will follow or the festivals they will celebrate, since these differ widely, depending on a person's region of origin, caste, family and sect, and on his or her individual choice.

This diversity can make Hinduism difficult for non-Hindus to understand. However, beneath the apparent diversity there is also a clear unity. There are certain fundamental truths and values which all, or almost all, devout Hindus would acknowledge. Among these are: the existence of one Supreme Spirit; the immortal soul that exists in all living things; the cycle of reincarnation; release from this cycle as the ultimate aim of life; karma, the natural cycle of reward and punishment for every act and thought; a clear code of dutiful and right behaviour; non-violence; and the supreme duty of seeking Truth.

Although there is great variation within Hindu practice and belief, for each individual his or her own religious beliefs and duties are clear. The variations may cause problems for people who try to define and describe Hinduism from the outside, but do not worry Hindus themselves.

Most Hindus feel it is very important to recognise that as human beings we can only see part of the truth, part of reality. Individuals must deal with this part of reality as they understand it. Sorting out who is right and who is wrong, or struggling towards precise theological definitions, is irrelevant. The important things are to live as virtuously as one can, to worship the Supreme Spirit, to do one's duty, and to strive towards greater understanding; not to battle with ideas that we can anyway never fully grasp since we are only human.

3. Where did most Hindus in Britain come from?

The families of most of the Hindus in Britain came from East Africa; some came directly from India.

Those from India came mainly from Gujarat State on the western coast, and a few from Punjab State (see Map 1).

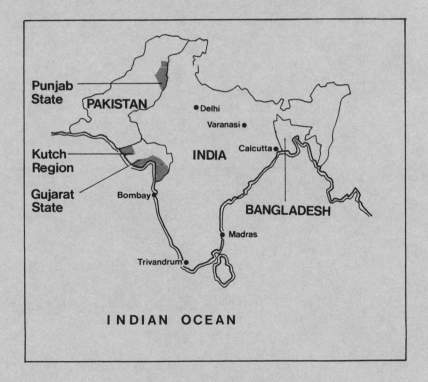

Map 1: The Indian subcontinent: showing the areas from which the main groups of Hindus came to Britain and went to East Africa.

The families of most Hindus from East Africa also originally emigrated from either Gujarat or Punjab, the majority again from Gujarat. Most of them settled in East Africa during the last hundred years. They came to Britain mainly from Kenya, Uganda and Tanzania, and also from Zambia and Malawi (see Map 2).

Gujaratis and Punjabis both have longstanding traditions of migration and travel: Gujaratis mainly as traders and

Table 1: *The main groups of Hindus in Britain*

Hindus from INDIA		
Mainly from	May be referred to as	First language
GUJARAT also from northern Gujarat; *Kutch* region	Gujarati Hindus Gujarati or Kutchi Hindus	Gujarati Gujarati or Kutchi (dialect of Gujarati)
PUNJAB	Punjabi Hindus	Punjabi or Hindi
also small groups from other areas: *e.g.* Delhi West Bengal Kerala Tamil Nadu	Bengali Hindus Kerala Hindus Tamil Hindus	Hindi or Punjabi Bengali Malayali Tamil
Hindus from EAST AFRICA		
Hindu families orginally emigrated Mainly from	May be referred to as	First language
GUJARAT	East African Gujarati Hindus	Gujarati
also from *Kutch* region in Northern Gujarat	East African Gujarati or Kutchi Hindus	Gujarati or Kutchi
Some from *PUNJAB*	East African Punjabi Hindus	Punjabi or Hindi
A few from *Delhi* and other areas		Hindi etc.

naval adventurers, and Punjabis in the army and other services.

Settlement in East Africa

At the time of Christ, Gujarati traders had already set up trading networks across the Indian Ocean in East Africa. These expanded over the centuries, and by the nineteenth century there were communities of Muslim and Hindu Gujarati traders living and trading in the towns along the East African coast, also becoming money lenders and financiers, administrators and customs collectors. Indian families settled in East Africa continued to maintain close links with their homes in India, travelling backwards and forwards and sending their children to and fro for education and marriage.

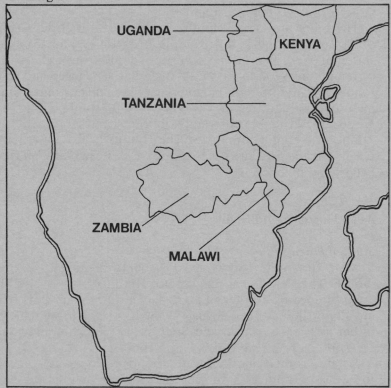

Map 2:   East Africa: showing the countries from which the main groups of Asians came to Britain

9

At the end of the nineteenth century the British colonised parts of East Africa and began to set up a formal colonial infrastructure in the interior. They imported manpower from India, initially to build a railway network, and then to maintain and service it and the settlements that grew up around it.

The British actively encouraged Indian immigration, recruiting people from Gujarat as artisans and clerks and as junior administrators in the government. Gujaratis and Punjabis also began to set up shops and businesses in East Africa.

The main settlement of Asian families in East Africa took place between 1890 and 1935, and, in a second period, between 1945 and 1960.

Other Hindu groups in Britain

There are also small Hindu communities in Britain from other areas of India, for example from Delhi, and from the states of West Bengal and Kerala. People from each of the different areas of India speak different languages and may follow certain different religious practices and customs. They may celebrate different festivals. Each Hindu group has tended to settle, worship and socialise separately in Britain.

Since the families of most of the Hindus in Britain originated in Gujarat and Punjab, this book focusses mainly on their beliefs and practices.

Asian languages in Britain

Spoken languages

Most Hindus in Britain speak Gujarati or Punjabi as their mother tongue. Some may speak Hindi, which is also the lingua franca of northern India. Gujarati, Punjabi and Hindi are all northern Indian languages, and have certain similarities, rather as French, Italian and Spanish do. Punjabi and Hindi are fairly close; so are Gujarati and Hindi.

Whatever their mother tongue, most people in northern India learn Hindi as a subject (as children in England learn French) in secondary school. Higher education is usually in Hindi. People from northern India with secondary or higher education are therefore likely to be able to communicate with each other to some extent in spoken Hindi, whatever their first language.

The languages spoken in southern India are from a completely different language family and have little in common with northern Indian languages. People from southern and northern India may have no common language. The lingua franca in southern India is English.

Written languages

Gujarati and Hindi are written in two very different forms of the Devanagri alphabet, and Punjabi is usually written in a related but different alphabet, Gurmukhi. Most people who speak several Indian languages, therefore, only read one. This is important when giving out leaflets or written material.

4. The Hindu world-view

The term Hinduism covers a large number of differing beliefs and religious practices. There are however certain central truths held by all, or almost all, who call themselves Hindu.

4.1 The Supreme Spirit

For Hindus there is one Ultimate Reality, one Supreme Spirit, from which the whole of the universe emanates. This Supreme Spirit or Super Consciousness is without form or name, without gender, without qualities or attributes. It is absolute and impersonal, infinite and all-pervading. It is beyond anything of which human beings can conceive or begin to imagine. It is also the essence and source of every possible virtue and form and of all life.

From this Ultimate Reality, this Supreme Spirit, comes the universe. From It all living things in the universe are drawn, and to It all will return. Only the Supreme Spirit is real and eternal, the Ultimate Reality; everything else, including this earth and its contents, is illusory and transitory. The Supreme Spirit also resides in every human being in the form of a soul or life force — atman. This soul will ultimately be released to merge with the Supreme Spirit. The final religious goal of all living things is to escape this illusory world through worship and devotion, and to be reunited with the Supreme Spirit, the Ultimate Reality, which is the only Truth. The Supreme Spirit may be known by many different names, for example, Brahman, Bhagwan, Parameshwar (Highest Lord), Paramatma (Supreme Spirit), Ishwar (Lord).

> I am the taste of living waters and the light of the sun and the moon. I am OM, the sacred word of the Vedas, sound in silence, heroism in men.

I am the pure fragrance that comes from the earth and the brightness of fire I am. I am the life of all living beings, and the austere life of those who train their souls.

And I am from everlasting the seed of eternal life. I am the intelligence of the intelligent. I am the beauty of the beautiful.

I am the power of those who are strong, when this power is free from passions and selfish desires. I am desire when this is pure, when this desire is not against righteousness.

Bhagavad Gita 7:8–11

Hindus believe that, because our mental, emotional and intuitive powers are human and therefore limited, we cannot begin to understand the Supreme Spirit which is Ultimate Reality. We need easier ways to approach and worship It. Consequently, Hindus worship the Supreme Spirit by focussing on the different aspects of the created universe in which It resides. Many of these aspects are personified and formalised as deities or gods. Whichever god one worships, one is always, consciously or unconsciously, worshipping the incomprehensible, the infinite, the Supreme Spirit, the Absolute.

Hindus categorise everything that happens in the world as creative, preserving, or destructive. These three aspects can be seen in all the cycles that we observe in nature and around us. Everything in the universe, whether small or large, is part of an eternal cycle; is growing or being created, is being maintained or preserved, or is decaying or dying.

These three major aspects are personified or symbolised in the three main Hindu gods: Brahma, the Creator, who symbolises creative power; Vishnu, the Preserver, who preserves and maintains what has been created; and Shiva, the Destroyer, who brings all things to an end. Each of these major aspects and the qualities inherent in them may be worshipped separately. They can also be personified and worshipped in other ways, for example as a human incarnation of a deity, such as Rama and Krishna; or as a female deity who represents worthwhile areas of human endeavour, such as Saraswati (or Knowledge), Lakshmi (or Prosperity), Amba (or the Benign Mother). There are also revered teachers or living saints who show the path of Truth and who influence people by their wisdom and those aspects of their character which are divine. All of the above may be worshipped as manifestations or aspects of the Ultimate Reality which we cannot fully understand.

When a man sees that the infinity of various beings is abiding in the ONE, and is an evolution from the ONE, then he becomes one with Brahman.

Bhagavad Gita 13:30

4.2 Reincarnation and karma

For Hindus, all living things in this world are subject to reincarnation; the cycle of birth, death, and rebirth in the material world. This cycle is called sansar. However, every living being also has an eternal soul or spirit, atman. This is part of and springs from the Supreme Spirit, which is often referred to as Paramatma. When any living thing dies, its immortal spirit, its atman, does not die. It is reborn in another body.

As a man leaves an old garment and puts on one that is new, the Spirit leaves his mortal body and then puts on one that is new.

Weapons cannot hurt the Spirit and fire can never burn him. Untouched is he by drenching waters, untouched is he by parching winds.

Bhagavad Gita 2:22—23

Where and in what condition one's spirit is reborn depends entirely on what one has done in previous lives, the ratio of good and evil deeds and attainments. In the same way each person's status, situation and good or ill fortune in this life are an investment in the future, and will be the direct cause of their status, situation and good or ill fortune in future lives. Every action inevitably has a result. This natural cycle of reward and punishment for all deeds and thoughts is called karma.

Belief in karma leads to a very strong and clear sense of personal responsibility. You know that you are responsible for what you are now, because what you are now is entirely a result of your past actions and thoughts. And you know that your actions and thoughts now will determine how you are born and your circumstances in your next life. Belief in karma may also affect people's reactions to, for example, illness and crisis, in that it may help to provide an understanding and an explanation for what has happened and, with it, a sense of resignation. Nothing is an accident. At the same time, Hindu belief stresses the importance of striving to do one's duty in any situation, and by so doing, to ensure good karma for the future. Belief in karma leads to acceptance but not to fatalism.

In a sense, karma is a doctrine combining total free will and total responsibility. You are the only person who is responsible for your condition now, and only you can determine your future.

Good karma, that is, happiness and security in this life and in the next, can be actively ensured through doing one's duty as prescribed by one's status; honouring and revering one's parents, the elderly, saints and priests; protecting the weak; disciplining one's desires; doing good to others and giving to the poor; providing hospitality to guests; performing prescribed religious ceremonies; following religious restrictions, for example, avoiding certain foods and fasting; pilgrimage, sacrifice, and worship.

Central to Hinduism is the belief that all things in the world are inter-linked, and that everything affects everything else: the movement of the stars and planets affects people, events, and natural phenomena on earth; bad and good occurrences affect nature and the stars and planets; prayer, sacrifice, pilgrimage and good deeds positively affect natural and human events and can change their course for the better; a person's every action or thought influences his or her future for better or for worse. Karmic forces operate in everything; everything is linked into the cycle of karma; nothing is unaffected.

Karma affects groups and nations and families as well as individuals; if people as a group do and think evil and are selfish and greedy, they inevitably sow evil for themselves and will reap only unhappiness and suffering in the future. Many devout Hindus point to this as exemplified in the state of the world today.

4.3 Release from the cycle of reincarnation
Hindus recognise that the cycle of birth, life and death in

this world — sansar — and of punishment and reward — karma — inevitably involve pain and suffering. The ultimate aim of all living things is therefore to be released from the cycle of endless births and earthly existence and to be reunited with the Supreme Spirit. This final release is called moksha. All Hindus believe in moksha — release — as an ultimate goal.

Moksha, release from the cycle of earthly existence, is extremely difficult to achieve. It can be achieved by ridding oneself of one's sense of ego, of the outward movement of the mind, and of one's attachment to the world and to worldly things, affections and obsessions. People may try to achieve this in different ways, for example, through subjecting themselves to extreme physical deprivation, giving up their home and family and wandering the world in renunciation; through praise and worship; or though learning.

For the vast majority of Hindus, however, trying to attain moksha in this life too difficult. Most Hindus, while recognising moksha is the ultimate goal of all living things, concentrate on living a good life in terms of this world: doing one's duty, doing good, and avoiding harm to any living thing. Although they will not reach moksha at the end of this life, they will be rewarded by good karma in the next, and so by the shortening of the cycle of birth, life and death.

Hindus believe that, just as all rivers, though they seem to flow in many directions, lead ultimately to one great ocean, so all ways and faiths, even unbelief, lead ultimately to Truth. Every human being is at a different stage of awareness and progress towards Truth; no method of worship or devotion is worse or better than any other.

4.4 Duty

The concept of duty — dharma — good and proper conduct, is very important in Hinduism. Most people do not aspire to moksha, unity with the Supreme Spirit, but concentrate on living a virtuous and dutiful life in this world, with the goal of achieving good karma in the next life.

Certain duties, very similar to those in other major religions, apply to everyone: to seek the truth, to reject evil in all its forms, to earn one's living righteously, to protect the weak, to discipline one's desires, and to revere life. As daily duties, every Hindu must pray and worship, show reverence to saints, priests, and teachers, honour and care for parents and elders, give hospitality to guests and strangers, give charity to the poor and needy, and conduct religious ceremonies at the appropriate times.

Depending on their social status, age and position in life, every Hindu also has certain other social and religious duties to perform; for example, certain behaviour is required of a brother or a child or a parent, a teacher or a farmer. Doing all one's duties as well as one can is usually considered more important and valuable than struggling to understand theological complexities.

> Greater is thine own work, even if this be humble, than the work of another, even if this be great. When a man does the work God gives him, no sin can touch this man.
>
> And a man should not abandon his work, even if he cannot achieve it in full perfection; because in all work there may be imperfection, even as in all fire there is smoke.
>
> *Bhagavad Gita* 18:47—48

People from higher castes are traditionally considered to be on a higher spiritual plane and so have greater religious duties and must follow stricter prohibitions than people from lower castes. They must pay more attention to avoiding spiritual and physical impurity. Devout Hindus from higher caste groups, for example, are likely to be more strict about what they eat, about not eating from utensils that have been used for non-vegetarian meals, and about bathing and praying in hospital.

4.5 Purity and impurity

The idea of purity and impurity is central to Hinduism, and to Hindu social structure and religious practice. For a Hindu, purity and impurity have both physical and spiritual aspects, and impurity has spiritual consequences. Certain everyday things, mainly to do with decay and death and bodily emissions, are intrinsically impure and are spiritually polluting. Purity should be ensured by avoiding or rapidly removing anything that is impure. Those who have been in contact with impurity must therefore purify themselves before returning to normal life and certainly before any act of worship or contact with sacred things. Running water is a particularly effective purifying agent. Many Hindu ceremonies concentrate on purification; fire is regarded as a symbol of purification and cleansing and is an important part of ceremonial worship.

The basic framework of purity and impurity has many consequences for personal and social behaviour and is shared by all Hindus, though there is a good deal of variation in how far individuals put it into practice. Bodily cleanliness is always extremely important; people will wish to wash or shower frequently. Food is ranked on a scale of purity, meat (dead flesh) being for most Hindus the most impure and defiling. Different jobs or tasks are in themselves considered more or less pure, and the people who perform these tasks are ranked accordingly in castes within Hindu society. The more pure groups or castes are traditionally considered worthy of respect from the less pure; they may avoid tasks, or contacts, or substances or sometimes even human contacts, which might make them less pure, and may be careful to maintain their higher state of spiritual purity.

The principles that underlie Hindu ideas of purity and pollution are completely different from Western notions of purity and hygiene, although views about what is and is not clean in the two traditions will often overlap. It is important to remember, however, that Hindu ideas about purity and impurity have religious force.

4.6 Respect for life

Hindus believe that the soul or life force – atman – in all living things is interconnected and that all living things are part of one great cycle of birth and rebirth. Some Hindus consider that only human beings and animals have a soul, others, for example, Jains, include insects and plants and everything that lives.

All living things, as part of the same cycle, are subject to the same laws; human beings are not more important in the scale of living things than animals and birds. All life, human and non-human, is sacred and must be treated with respect. This contrasts with traditional Christian, Jewish and Muslim belief in which human beings are unique, in that only they have souls, and animals and other living things are beings of a lesser order, with no eternal soul, placed on earth largely for the service of humanity. Belief in the sacredness of life is part of the basis of Hindu vegetarianism; human beings do not have the right to kill or misuse any other living creature for their own purposes. The Hindu doctrine of ahimsa, or non-violence, therefore applies not only to other people, but to all living creatures.

> He who sees that the Lord of all is ever the same in all that is, immortal in the field of mortality — he sees the truth.
> And when a man sees that the God in himself is the same God in all that is, he hurts not himself by hurting others: then he goes indeed to the highest Path.
>
> *Bhagavad Gita* 13:27–28

Precise interpretations of ahimsa vary: Jains, for example, whose religion, Jainism, is a development of Hinduism, generally thought to have been founded in or before the sixth century B.C., believe that all living things, including beings too small for us to see, are part of the great cycle of birth and rebirth. In India very devout Jains sweep the ground before them to avoid treading on and harming any small living thing. Members of one Jains sect cover their mouths with gauze to avoid breathing in any living thing.

4.7 The Hindu deities

Most Hindus worship the Supreme Spirit, the Ultimate Reality, through a symbol or manifestation, a male or female deity.

There are many different Hindu gods and goddesses, each with different qualities and characters. Pictures or statues of them may be seen in Hindu homes and temples. Vishnu, Shiva and Brahma (see 4.1 above) are normally regarded as the three main gods. Most people worship Vishnu or Shiva, either directly or through another manifestation or an incarnation. Many people focus their main worship on a female deity or principle. She too may be worshipped under many different names and in many different guises. She may be called, for example, Shakti (energy), Devi (goddess), or Mataji (mother goddess), and is particularly powerful in her own right. Most male gods also have a female counterpart, a goddess, the two complementing each other to form a balanced whole. The three main gods, Vishnu, Shiva and Brahma, are usually depicted with Lakshmi, Parvati and Saraswati as their consorts, but, again, these goddesses may take different forms.

Often the same god or goddess is worshipped under different names in the different parts of India. The gods and goddesses are, like humans, subject to the cycle of birth and rebirth, and to the forces of karma. The stories of the gods and goddesses form Hindu mythology, and form part of the environment in which a Hindu child grows up and through which it learns its values and beliefs.

Which god or gods a person worships depends on their area of origin, family tradition and on personal choice. Certain additional local or village or personal gods may be particularly worshipped at certain times or for certain favours. Hindu family shrines and temples usually contain statues or symbols of different gods. Individuals may worship one or several. Each is represented in such a way as to symbolise his or her particular qualities:

Major deities (details and names vary a good deal in different parts of India and between individuals)

Brahma, Creative Power, is usually represented with four heads to indicate that he controls all four corners of the universe. He often rides a gander, which symbolises knowledge, the vehicle of each god being a manifestation of his powers in an animal form. The breathing of the gander represents the life breath of the whole universe. Brahma is known to all Hindus but is rarely, if ever, worshipped himself.

His consort is Saraswati, goddess of learning and the arts, of wisdom and of music.

Vishnu represents permanence, continuity and preservation. At times of injustice and moral chaos Vishnu is born into the world as an incarnation to conquer evil and to reteach human beings the moral code they have forgotten or ignored. Vishnu has already been incarnated nine times in this world in different forms, and will come again for the last time when evil and disorder threaten mankind again. Vishnu rides Garuda,

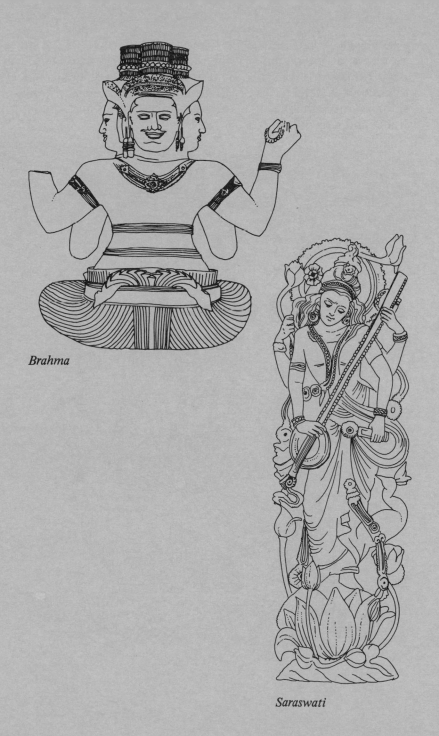

Brahma

Saraswati

21

a sun-eagle, that kills snakes and conquers evil. One of Vishnu's sacred symbols is the tulsi plant, a form of basil. People may grow a tulsi plant in their home or garden in honour of Vishnu. Vishnu is usually represented and worshipped through one of his human incarnations or avatars, Rama and Krishna.

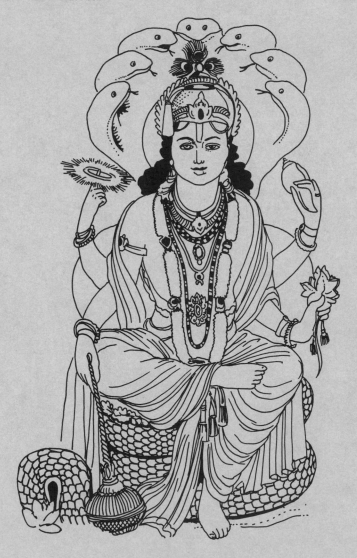

Vishnu's consort is Lakshmi, the goddess of good fortune, success and prosperity. She is the embodiment of female beauty. She is often represented with four arms to show her great power and skill. She is worshipped at the festival of Diwali, and there are pictures and statues of her in many homes and over the door of Hindu temples.

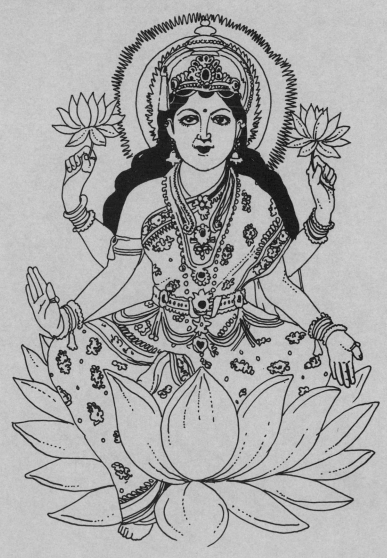

Lakshmi

Shiva, also known as Shankar and Mahadev, is worshipped in many forms and manifestations. He has a third eye in the centre of his forehead which he opens to destroy the world when it has been overtaken by evil. Shiva maintains the continual ebb and flow and dissolution and recreation of the world and of the universe by his dance. Shiva is also regarded as the giver of sexual fertility. In temples and shrines he is often represented by a stone symbol, the lingam.

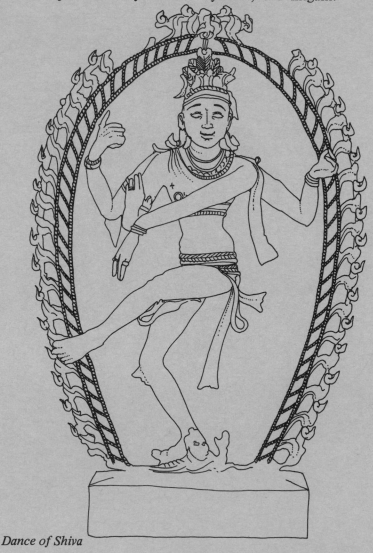

Dance of Shiva

Shiva's consort is Parvati, who is worshipped under many names and in many forms. As Durga, the Unapproachable, she rides a lion and has eight hands to wield the weapons of the gods.

Incarnations of Vishnu

Krishna is the eighth avatar (incarnation) of Vishnu. He and Rama, the seventh avatar, are the gods most generally worshipped by Hindus in Britain.

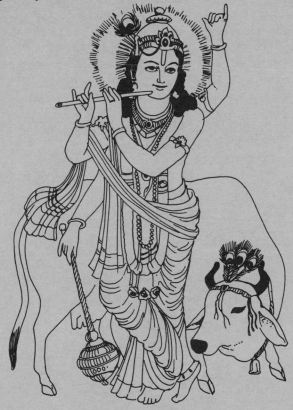

Krishna

The story of Krishna's life is told in the epic poem, the Mahabharata. The most beloved of all Hindu texts, the Bhagavad Gita, contains the words of Krishna on good and evil, duty and devotion, faith and salvation. Many Hindus in Britain pray to Krishna as their supreme deity. He is often depicted with blue skin.

Krishna's consort is Radha, whom some regard as an incarnation of the goddess Lakshmi (the consort of Vishnu).

Rama is the seventh avatar (incarnation) of Vishnu and, like Krishna, because he is both human and divine, is a focus of worship and devotion for many Hindus. His heroic deeds are told in the other major Hindu epic, the Ramayana. The Ramayana is told in different languages all over India, and contains parables and allegories and stories full of meaning for all Hindus. In it Rama's wife Sita (an incarnation of Lakshmi) is kidnapped by Ravana, the evil king of Lanka. Rama finally rescues her with the help of the monkey god Hanuman. The rescue of Sita symbolises the victory of good over evil. Many Hindus worship Rama as their supreme deity and Rama and Sita are often regarded as a model for all married couples.

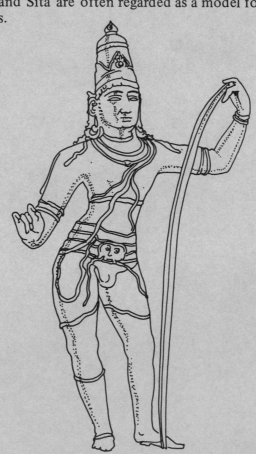

Rama

Other deities

Other lesser deities may be worshipped by some people or may be worshipped at particular times for their special qualities:

Ganesh is the son of Shiva and his consort Parvati. He is represented with four arms and an elephant's head. Ganesh is the god of wisdom and because of his wisdom and strength can remove all obstacles and make all ventures succeed. He is regarded as symbolising helping qualities. Most Hindus have an image of Ganesh in their homes for protection and good fortune. Ganesh is invoked and worshipped at the beginning of any new undertaking, such as a business venture, a course of study, or a wedding. His symbol 卐 indicates good luck and purity and may be seen in Hindu homes and temples.

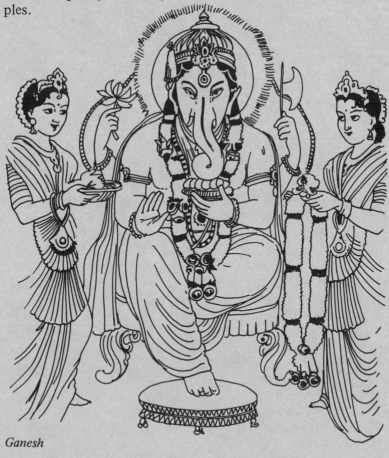

Ganesh

Hanuman is represented as a monkey. In the Ramayana he helps Rama, the seventh incarnation of Vishnu, to rescue his wife Sita. For his services he is granted immortality. He symbolises the ideal of selfless and devoted service to a master, which Hindus should emulate in their worship and lives.

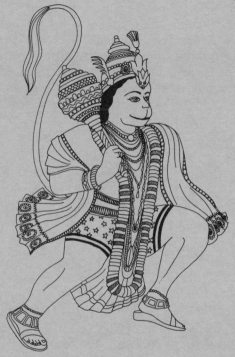

Hanuman

Hindus in Britain

Most Hindus in Britain are Vaishnavs, that is, their worship focusses mainly on Vishnu, often in the form of his incarnation, Krishna. At the same time, people also accept other gods, as each having different qualities, a different personality, and a different role to play. They may have statues or pictures of other gods in their homes or in the temple, and may worship them at particular times of the year, or on particular occasions such as at the beginning of a new enterprise. Certain festivals are devoted to particular gods, for example, Janmastami, in August or September, celebrates the birth of Krishna; Diwali, in October or November, is in honour of the goddess Lakshmi.

28

5. The Hindu holy books

Hindus have many holy writings. The oldest, the four Vedas (Veda means knowledge), were compiled between four and five thousand years ago and are regarded as sacred and immortal revelations. The Vedas are written in Sanskrit, an ancient Indo-European language. They discuss the nature and purpose of human existence and of the world. They also contain legends about the gods, hymns, and rules for the conduct of religious ceremonies. Nowadays the Vedas are mainly used in religious ceremonies.

The Upanishads, also written in Sanskrit, date from between 500 and 200 B.C. and are also regarded as sacred revelations. They discuss the relationship of the human soul with the Supreme Spirit.

The two great Hindu epic poems, the Ramayana and the Mahabharata, are told in slightly differing versions and in all the different languages all over India. They were written between 300 B.C. and A.D. 30. Both poems discuss, through the heroic episodes which they relate, human nature and moral values; each episode casts light on human dilemmas and duties, and stories from the two epics form the basis of many Hindu folk tales, and of much proverbial wisdom.

For Hindus, the Ramayana, about Rama, the seventh incarnation of Vishnu, and the Mahabharata, about Krishna, the eighth incarnation of Vishnu, perform the same kinds of function as the Old Testament for Christians and Jews: history, allegory, guidance, proverbs, stories with a message, insight into unchanging aspects of human nature and the battle between good and evil. Many people have copies of the Ramayana and the Mahabharata in their homes.

The Bhagavad Gita
The most loved and widely read of all Hindu Holy Books is

the Bhagavad Gita, sometimes known as the Gita. It is an excerpt from the Mahabharata.

In the Gita, Krishna, a human incarnation of Vishnu, teaches that each person must love and worship the Supreme Spirit and must do to the best of their ability what their station demands of them; they must devote themselves self-lessly to this sacred duty with no thought of personal gain. Each person's duty and role in the world, and each person's ability and spiritual awareness are different, and must be accepted as such. Each person must do their duty without fear or favour, out of a sense of duty and without expectation of reward.

Patients may bring a copy of the Gita into hospital with them. Like any sacred Hindu text, it must be kept clean and safe, and is usually wrapped in a cotton or silk cloth for protection. It should not be put on the floor or near the feet, and nothing should be put on top of it. People should be clean and wash their hands before they read the Bhagavad Gita or other holy books.

The Bhagavad Gita is revered and loved by all Hindus, with much the same attitude as devout Christians have for the New Testament. Parts of the Bhagavad Gita are read to children by their mothers, recited at ceremonies, read at cremations, and read by many as part of their daily morning prayer. The Bhagavad Gita may be used to swear in Hindu witnesses in a British court of law. Many Hindu parents are most concerned that their children growing up in this country should learn to read their mother tongue so that they can read the Bhagavad Gita and other religious books.

Hindus, like Christians, may also read other prayer books, devotional writings, and stories of holy people. These are most likely to be in Hindi or in the mother tongue of most of the Hindus in Britain, either Gujarati or Punjabi. Any religious books brought into hospital should be treated with respect.

6. Hindu worship

Hindu worship (puja) is essentially individual, though some Hindu sects stress congregational worship. Most people worship at home but many people also like to go to the temple (mandir) to worship. In Britain, where Hindu temples are often few and far between and are not open all day, people may find it more difficult to visit the temple.

6.1 Worship at home

Most Hindu homes contain a small shrine where family members can worship. This may be in a separate room, or, if there is not enough space, it may be set up in a corner or in a small glass-fronted cabinet. How regularly people worship depends on family tradition, personal devotion and opportunity. Very devout Hindus may pray three times a day; at sunrise, around noon, and at sunset. It is most important to purify oneself by washing before praying. A devout Hindu should always take a shower and perform puja (pray) before eating or drinking in the morning.

In Hindu tradition women are chiefly responsible for ensuring that the family's religious duties are carried out, for the religious education and guidance of children, and for handing down family traditions of worship. In Britain, where most people have busy routines, the women may say the prayers for the whole family.

The exact details of each family shrine will differ, but there are usually statues (murti) of one or more gods particularly worshipped by the family, and pictures and prints of others and of saints revered by the family. There may also be incense sticks to create a pleasant and sweet-smelling atmosphere. People may put flowers on the shrine and also small symbolic offerings of food. Sometimes the shrine is in the kitchen, the purest and cleanest place in the house since it is the place where food is prepared.

> He who offers to me with devotion only a leaf, or a flower, or a fruit, or even a little water, this I accept from that yearning soul, because with a pure heart it was offered with love.
>
> *Bhagavad Gita* 9:26

If a family has a separate room for their shrine this must be kept pure and should not be entered without an invitation. Anyone who enters must take off their shoes. Women may be asked to cover their heads. No one should touch anything on a shrine unless specifically invited to.

At special times Hindu families may organise a hawan. This is a special ceremony of purification in which fire is used to symbolise purifying force. A hawan is performed, for example, at a marriage, after a birth, to celebrate and give thanks for a special event, or when someone has died. The ceremony itself is performed by a pandit — priest — and may be held in the family home, rather like a Roman Catholic family mass, or in a community hall. Relatives and close friends are invited to the ceremony.

6.2 Worship in hospital

Worship and prayer in hospital are matters for individual decision. Ask Hindu patients whether they will need any special facilities and whether there are times at which they will not wish to be disturbed.

Some devout Hindus may wish to pray in the morning before they eat or drink. It is important to purify oneself by showering or washing before praying. Bedbound patients may need help with this. A sponge-bath should be given if possible. If not, at least patients should be able to wash their hands and sprinkle clean water over their heads to symbolise washing.

Some people may wish to sit up cross-legged on the bed to pray or to read holy books, rather than remain lying down. (Hindus do not usually kneel to pray.) A few patients may set up a small shrine in front of them with a picture or statue on it. People may say prayers, repeat holy phrases — mantras

— read a passage from a holy book, or merely sit and meditate. Some Hindus may use a mala — a string of beads — to aid their concentration while they recite. A mala must be touched with clean hands and treated with reverence. It may be kept in a small cloth bag. People should obviously not be disturbed while praying.

Hindu patients may also wish to pray around midday and in the evening. As in the morning, they will usually want to wash first. Some people may wish to draw the curtains round their bed while praying; some cover their heads with a scarf or a piece of cloth.

Patients or their visitors may also wish to recite prayers or sing hymns quietly. They may like to draw the curtains round the bed or to use a side-ward if one is available.

In some cases families will wish to perform special religious ceremonies for someone who is ill, for example, praying, reciting hymns, and blessing the sick person with water or tying a symbolic thread round one arm. These ceremonies are usually simple and can easily be accommodated on a ward, though some people may prefer a side-ward for privacy. Some families choose to perform these special ceremonies at home for someone who is sick in hospital, so as to avoid embarrassment and disturbance to ward routines.

6.3 Worship at the temple

Hindus may also go to a temple — mandir — to worship. In Britain, the mandir may be particularly important as a place where people of the same community can meet.

Some people, generally the elderly and women who do not go to work, attend the mandir every day if they can. Some people may go to the mandir in the evenings after work. Most families, however, only attend on major festivals, and on Sundays, to fit in best with British routines.

No one should enter the mandir unless they are pure and physically clean. Everyone must remove their shoes and women must cover their heads.

In the mandir there are usually statues and pictures of several gods with one in a central position, depending on the preferences of the congregation. The whole congregation sits on the floor, usually men and older boys on one side, women, girls and very young children on the other.

People pray individually before the deities, often bowing or kneeling as a sign of reverence. They may lean forward to touch the shrine and then their head and body to transfer some of the divinity of the god to themselves. Sometimes there is congregational singing of hymns — bhajans — to a particular deity, while a priest performs the necessary rituals.

Almost every mandir in Britain has a resident Brahmin priest — a pandit — appointed and paid by the congregation to perform the prescribed everyday ceremonies, to tend the shrines of the gods, and to perform special ceremonies at festivals or at the request of a particular family. Formal Hindu ceremonies must always be performed by Brahmins, people from the highest Hindu caste, who are considered to be spiritually purer and higher and to have a special religious role enabling them to interpret the deity to the congregation. The pandit acts as an intermediary between the worshipper and the deity.

In the early days of Hindu settlement in Britain it was often difficult for a community to get a Brahmin priest, since devout high caste Hindus traditionally believed that it was spiritually defiling to leave the soil of India. Now, however, attitudes have changed and it is easier to find pandits who will come to Britain. Many pandits come over for only a short period, for example two or three years, to work in a particular mandir and then return home to their families in India. Not all of them speak English.

Hindu congregations in Britain may also invite visiting preachers — swamis — to come and teach them at the temple. Swamis with special reputations may be invited to come from India.

Each mandir is run by an elected committee from the local community. The committee is usually headed by a President and a Secretary. The best way to make contact with a local Hindu temple is usually through the Secretary. Non-Hindu visitors are usually made very welcome at a mandir.

Teachers

Any great or good person may be seen as a partial incarnation of the divine. Many Hindus, for example, regard both Christ and Gandhi as having divine qualities.

Religious teachers (gurus) of special sanctity may also be worshipped. They are regarded as particularly close to an understanding of the Truth, and as channels or guides through whom ordinary people may reach greater understanding and insight. Many Hindus have personal gurus who may lay down particular rules and spiritual and physical disciplines for their followers or may write books of spiritual guidance and meditation.

6.4 Pilgrimage

Like members of other religions, Hindus may go on pilgrimages to holy places.

Many Hindus believe that by performing a religious pilgrimage they will gain special blessings for themselves and for their families.

People may also sometimes make a pilgrimage for a special cause, for example, to be cured of a disease, to ensure a successful pregnancy after several miscarriages, or for a sick member of the family.

Some travel agents in Britain in areas of Hindu settlement organise package tours to centres of pilgrimage in India.

The most holy place of all to Hindus is Varanasi (also known as Benares) on the sacred River Ganga (Ganges). Varanasi is particularly sacred to worshippers of Shiva and of Rama. Elderly people may wish to go to Varanasi so that they may die in a holy place. After a Hindu is cremated his or her ashes may be taken to India to be scattered on the waters of the River Ganga, particularly at Varanasi. Pilgrims who have been to Varanasi often bring home a bottle of water from the Ganga which they may place on the family shrine. They may place drops of this holy water in the mouth of someone who is dying.

7. Hindu families

7.1 Family duties

The family is central to Hindu life and to Hindu communities as it is to all communities from the Indian subcontinent. In Asian culture the family is traditionally a much larger unit, often referred to as the extended family, and includes people whom most British people would regard as distant relatives. For most Hindus in Britain obligations to family members in India and in East Africa remain very strong.

Hindus are expected to marry, and both men and women are expected to take an active part in bringing up children. There is a very strict code of sexual morality to protect families and communities. Premarital and extramarital sex are strictly forbidden. Deep shame follows the discovery of illicit liaisons, and this may affect the whole extended family.

Some Hindu families from East Africa may bring up their children with a greater degree of social freedom and independence than Hindu families from India. Ideas about sexual morality are still however likely to be extremely strict, and family bonds will generally remain strong.

Parents remain responsible for their children all their lives. Children are considered to have a debt to their parents which they should repay by obedience, by caring for them when they are old, and by marrying and bringing up their own family well. Showing respect and caring for one's elders are religious duties for Hindus.

When a relative is ill all family members have strong and unavoidable duties. Everyone who can must visit a sick relative in hospital or at home to give comfort and support. Anyone who does not is regarded as callous and very discourteous. Female relatives will often take over the care of a child if its own mother is sick. If an older relative back in India or East Africa is ill, family members may go at very short notice to look after them for long periods of time.

7.2 The roles of men and women

In traditional Hindu society, particularly in rural areas, the roles of men and women are clearly distinguished: men are in overall authority and are responsible for all matters outside the home and for supporting their families; women are responsible for rearing and educating children, looking after the family, and for running the home. These roles of course increasingly overlap in changing modern society. However, one of women's most important duties is to teach children and grandchildren about their religion and to teach them moral and religious values. Women are still regarded as in many senses the custodians of family values and morals, including religious traditions and practices. This is particularly important because the family (rather than formal religious organisations) is the main channel through which Hindu beliefs and values are handed down. The traditions of each family have a great influence on, for example, the deities that family members worship and the religious practices they follow.

As in Asian tradition generally, sons are considered responsible for the care and support of their parents as they grow older. This contrasts strongly with traditional British patterns. In Asian tradition, when a son marries he and his wife often remain with his parents and bring up their children there. In Britain, with smaller houses and greater job mobility, this is often more difficult, but at least one son and his family, usually the oldest, will generally try to remain with his parents. The oldest son in a Hindu family also has the specific religious duty of lighting his father's funeral pyre. This is regarded as very important, and a Hindu father with no son to perform this crucial duty is considered extremely unlucky.

Within most families, although men are considered to have ultimate authority, men and women generally share decisions. Women, as mentioned, are traditionally chiefly responsible for the comfort of their families, the upbringing and moral education of the children, and the atmosphere and conduct of the home. One of the traditional religious duties of a Hindu woman is to honour and obey her husband. In turn

Hinduism stresses that husbands must treat their wives with kindness and respect. Women are particularly honoured when they become mothers.

Relationships between men and women in Hindu families in Britain will obviously vary a good deal depending on factors such as age, educational background, whether women go out to work, and the length of time that the family has lived in Britain. Older members in all families will generally expect more traditional relationships and behaviour.

As among Muslims and Sikhs, there is a strong Hindu code of etiquette which is likely to influence behaviour between the sexes in public. Traditional female virtues such as decorum and modesty remain important to most Hindu women. In Asian cultural tradition men and women do not mix socially and are generally segregated from puberty. This is likely to be retained to some extent in Britain.

7.3 The elderly

The role of the elderly is well defined in Hinduism. Elderly people are revered and it is the absolute duty of all younger members of the family to support and obey them. All younger people are expected to behave respectfully towards them.

It is considered correct, in Hindu tradition, that as people become older they should withdraw and concentrate more and more on spiritual matters and on prayer and meditation, leaving financial and other responsibilities to younger family members. They may become, for example, more strict about what they eat and more concerned about avoiding any impurity. They may wish to pray in private and undisturbed. Older Hindus may therefore find life in a British hospital or residential institution very difficult.

8. Practical care

Hindu men and women should be modest about their bodies. Many conservative Hindus find any exposure shocking and offensive; co-operation and thought may be required from staff in hospitals and other institutions to avoid causing unnecessary embarrassment and distress, and to preserve people's modesty during medical and nursing procedures.

8.1 Women

Hindu women should traditionally cover their legs, breasts and upper arms. For a conservative Hindu woman to uncover her legs may be as horrifying and humiliating as for an English woman to be required to walk around in public with her breasts exposed. Backless hospital gowns and garments that leave the legs bare or have a low neckline are immodest for conservative Hindu women, particularly in the presence of strangers, especially of strange men. Long hospital dressing gowns should be provided where possible.

Most women do not expect to undress fully except when they are alone. In the subcontinent women do not usually undress for a physical examination but uncover only parts of themselves at a time. This procedure may avoid distress for conservative Hindu women in Britain.

Clothes

Most Hindu women wear a sari over a blouse and underskirt. A sari is a length of material usually about 5 or 6 metres long. The midriff may sometimes, though not always, be left bare.

Hindu women of Punjabi origin may wear shalwar kameez instead of a sari. The kameez (shirt) is a long tunic with long or half sleeves. The shalwar are loose trousers. The width of the shalwar legs varies according to fashion particularly among younger women. With the shalwar kameez goes a long scarf called a chuni or dupatta which should traditionally cover the head and breasts. Older women and many married women will pull one end of the dupatta or chuni, or the end of the sari, over their head as a sign of respect and modesty in front of strangers, older people or men.

Many Hindu women and older girls who wear Western dress always wear trousers or long skirts to ensure that their legs are covered.

Saris and shalwar kameez are normally worn as both day and night wear. They are worn loose at night for comfort. Asian women coming into hospital should be informed that they may continue to wear their normal nightclothes if they prefer. For many women a sari or shalwar kameez is both more comfortable than a nightdress and avoids embarrassment over showing the legs or arms in public. Buying British-style nightdresses specially for a stay in hospital is sometimes done but is an unnecessary expense. Check what a woman would prefer to wear.

Hindu widows traditionally wear white, the colour of withdrawal from the world, with no jewellery or makeup.

Jewellery and makeup

When a Hindu woman marries she usually receives wedding jewellery. Most women are given a mangal sutra by their husbands or in-laws. This is a brooch, generally gold, strung on a necklace of gold or black beads. It is regarded as very precious and is not removed while a woman's husband lives. To remove it unnecessarily may cause great distress and worry. If problems arise, discuss them with the patient herself or her family.

Women may also receive other wedding jewellery, particularly gold. Most women receive a number of glass or gold wedding bangles. These should not be removed and real distress may be caused if they break or are forcibly removed. Some women wear one or more wedding rings. Unlike English wedding rings these often contain precious stones. Some women may wear gold or silver rings on their toes. Others may wear a small jewel on their nose. Wedding jewellery should not be removed unless absolutely necessary and in hospital should be taped like an English wedding ring if at all possible. If wedding jewellery is removed or broken this may upset a Hindu woman as much as the loss of a wedding ring would upset most English women. If an important item of jewellery must be removed, explain the reason and discuss this with the patient or her family first, to avoid causing distress.

Bindi/tilak

Many Hindu women wear a small coloured spot made of a quick-drying liquid on their foreheads. This is called a bindi (Gujarati: chandlo) and traditionally indicates that a woman is married. It is now also worn as makeup by some unmarried women. The bindi is generally red but may vary in colour to match the clothes. Widows do not wear a bindi.

A woman who has participated in a religious ceremony may wear a tilak, also a spot on the forehead, but traditionally made of saffron, rice charcoal or sandalwood and put on her forehead by the priest.

Hair parting

Many married Hindu women, particularly in the early years of their marriage or on special occasions or festivals, paint a red streak of vermilion powder (sindur) into the parting of their hair as a sign of their married status. This is sometimes put on for the first time by the bridegroom at the wedding ceremony. Some married women in Britain are embarrassed to wear sindur in their partings because of the attention it attracts.

Some Hindu women in hospital may want to apply their bindi and sindur fresh every morning.

Other jewellery and makeup

Hindu women may also wear other jewellery and makeup. Much of this may have important religious or cultural significance. For example, a woman may wear a medallion with a picture of her personal god or guru around her neck or arm; she may wear jewellery containing a particular protective gemstone; or a special blessed amulet around her arm or body which she has been given to prevent or cure certain illnesses or symptoms, or to ensure a safe delivery.

A woman in her first pregnancy may be given a gold bangle by her husband's sister at a ceremony during the seventh month. This is to ensure a successful pregnancy and safe delivery and must not be removed.

No jewellery should be removed without the permission of the patient or her family. If problems over jewellery or makeup arise these should be discussed beforehand in order to arrive at a solution acceptable to everyone. Most people are very happy to explain the significance of a particular item of jewellery to a sympathetic enquirer.

8.2 Men

Hindu men should cover themselves from the waist to the knees; nudity, even in the presence of other men, may be offensive.

Men's clothes

Most Indian men wear a Western-style shirt and trousers but some may wear traditional dress to relax in at home. This will usually be a kameez — a loose shirt with or without a collar — and trousers with a drawstring — pajama — or a dhoti. A dhoti is 5 or 6 metres of cloth, usually white, wrapped around the waist and drawn between the legs. Older men may wear pajama and a shirt with a high collar and buttons down the front — a kurta — or a longer coat — an achkan. Men in hospital will usually wear Western-style pyjamas or traditional pajama. (The word pajama originated in India.)

Religious jewellery
Sacred thread

Men and older boys of higher castes may wear a sacred thread — janeu — a white cotton thread with three strands, worn over the right shoulder and round the body. This is given to a Hindu boy at a religious ceremony to mark his admission to adulthood and to adult religious responsibilities. It is worn both during the day and at night and must be kept clean. It is changed for a fresh thread if it becomes dirty and at Hindu New Year. It should never be removed. A Hindu man is cremated still wearing his sacred thread. From a health worker's point of view, a Hindu man who wears a sacred thread is more likely to observe religious restrictions strictly.
Necklace

Men of some Hindu sects, for example, the Swami Narayan sect, may wear a bead necklace. Some Swami Narayan men may also wear a red spot — tika or bhai doot — on their foreheads. Other Hindu men may wear a tika on certain special occasions, and after religious ceremonies.

Other jewellery

Like a Hindu woman, a Hindu man may wear other jewellery with religious or cultural significance. He may wear a medallion with a picture of his personal god or guru around his neck or arm; he may wear a ring containing a special gemstone to cure or prevent illness or an amulet chosen and blessed by a priest or a guru. Again, no jewellery should be removed without permission from the patient or his family. Any problems should be discussed so that a solution acceptable to everyone can be reached.

8.3 Washing and purity

Much of traditional Hindu religious practice involves the removal or avoidance of any physical impurity or pollution. It may be particularly important to be aware of this in hospital, where so much activity revolves around physical care. All physical emanations from the body are considered polluting; urine, faeces, saliva, menstrual blood, mucus, sweat and semen.

Most Hindus are extremely careful to wash or shower frequently to get rid of any physical impurities. Running water is a particularly effective purifying agent, and most people prefer to shower, pouring water over themselves in a bowl, rather than bathe. Many Asian people find the idea of sitting in one's own bath water most disgusting. Where showers are not provided people may prefer to stand in the bath and use a small bowl to pour water over themselves. In British-style bathrooms this may cause problems with water splashing onto the floor.

Most Hindus also wash themselves with running water after using the lavatory. The left hand only is used for this purpose; the right hand is kept pure for handling food and other clean things. If no tap is provided in the cubicle, people normally take water for washing into the lavatory in a special jug or bottle. In British-style lavatories this may cause problems with water splashing onto the floor. Lavatory paper is not traditionally used in the subcontinent and may be regarded with distaste, though most Asian people in Britain use lavatory paper as well as water. Find out from patients whether they have or need a small jug with which to carry water into the lavatory. Where bidets are provided in the lavatory cubicle this will not be necessary.

Some people may clean out their nasal passages with water and spit out any phlegm, particularly when they wash first thing in the morning. Handkerchiefs may be considered disgusting since after blowing one's nose one carries the mucas around on one's person. Some people may wish to clean their tongue as well as their teeth. A metal or plastic tongue scraper is usually used. Some will also wish to rinse out their mouths after a meal. Bedbound patients may ask for a glass of water and a bowl into which they can rinse out their mouths.

Hinduism also emphasises the importance of purifying one-self and being physically clean in preparation for worship. Most people take a shower first thing in the morning before they pray. The do not eat or drink anything until they have washed and prayed. In hospital a devout Hindu may wish to shower or at least have a good wash before saying any prayers or reading holy scriptures. People who are bedbound or find it difficult to walk may wish for help with washing at certain times of the day before they pray. Older Hindus are particularly likely to feel that this is important.

The head is often considered to be a sacred part of the body and the hair should be washed frequently. People may also rub oil into their hair to keep it healthy and shiny.

The feet are the dirtiest part of the body: shoes are considered particularly polluting and should not be put with other possessions, for example in a bag with other clothes, or on a locker. Holy books and items should not be put on the floor or near someone's feet on a bed.

Not everyone will be equally concerned about purity and pollution but many devout Hindus will feel very strongly about keeping clean and avoiding any impurity, particularly when they are ill and away from home. People in hospital who feel dirty and polluted may be extremely distressed, particularly if they are bedbound and cannot wash themselves or if adequate washing and showering facilities are not available. It is important to be alert to this and to discuss any particular needs and wishes with patients or their relatives.

8.4 Menstruation and birth

According to traditions of purity and pollution, Hindu women are considered unclean during menstruation and for forty days after giving birth. They do not touch the family shrine, go to the temple, pray or touch holy books. They do not have sexual intercourse.

After childbirth, some women may stay indoors resting for the full forty days, not going out at all. In some cases this may affect attendance at postnatal and other clinics.

At the end of the period of uncleanness women normally take a special shower and clean themselves, their clothes and their room thoroughly. They then return to normal life.

Some conservative Hindu women do not cook while they are menstruating or during forty days after giving birth. It may however be impossible to stick to this tradition in Britain where there may be no other women to help look after the family.

As in many European traditions, Asian women may consider themselves physically vulnerable at these times. They may avoid anything that could give them a chill, such as showering or washing their hair, particularly in the cold British climate.

9. Hindu dietary restrictions

Many Hindus in Britain follow dietary restrictions, though there is a good deal of variation. In general, older people, women, and people who are more devout are most likely to be careful about what they eat. In addition, there are certain Hindu sects whose members are particularly strict about following food prohibitions.

Hindus whose families originated in Gujarat are particularly likely to follow a vegetarian diet. Most of what is said below applies to them. Some East African Hindus may be less strict than those Hindus who have come to Britain directly from India. Many, however, continued to follow dietary restrictions in East Africa.

Some Hindus in Britain from southern or eastern areas of India, most of whom are doctors, lawyers, and other professionals, may adhere less strictly to religious food restrictions. This should not, however, be taken for granted, since many come from high caste Hindu families and are likely to be very careful about their diet.

9.1 A vegetarian diet

Hindus believe that all forms of life are interdependent, and that all living things are sacred. Most Hindus feel that they do not have the right to take the life of another living creature just to sustain their own life, particularly when so many other foods are readily available. Consequently, most devout Hindus do not eat any food that has involved the taking of life, and meat may also be considered polluting. Many Hindus eat a vegetarian diet.

However, Hinduism does not have a central authoritative set of regulations, and so, within a general ideal of vegetarianism, different sects, families and individuals make their own decisions on what they can and cannot eat. Although these decisions are individual, they are not flexible. A strict vegetarian Hindu who eats meat, fish, eggs or meat products, even unknowingly, is likely to feel revolted and also polluted.

In hospital it will be necessary to find out from each patient what they do and do not eat and to make provision accordingly.

Meat and fish

Most Hindus do not eat meat, fish or anything made from them.

The cow is a sacred animal to Hindus. It is considered a symbol of the gentleness and unselfish love and giving of a mother, the antithesis of violence and greed. For these reasons the cow is protected and worshipped and the eating of beef is particularly strictly prohibited. The cow is also revered as a provider of milk and dairy products, essential to the survival of rural communities in India. To most devout Hindus, to kill a cow would be a grave sin demanding severe spiritual and physical penalties.

Some Hindus in Britain, mainly men, will eat certain kinds of meat. However, many Hindus who eat other meat still do not eat beef for the reasons given above. They may also not eat pork. The pig, like the rat in Britain, is a scavenging animal in India and is considered unclean. Processed pork foods may be more acceptable to some people.

Non-vegetarian Hindus may eat fish, especially the white (non-oily) varieties.

Eggs

Eggs are potentially a source of life. In Asian tradition they are therefore not a vegetarian food. Many normal British vegetarian dishes, such as egg salads and omelettes, are not acceptable to strict Hindu vegetarians. Hindu men are more likely to eat eggs than women.

Unfertilised battery eggs are not literally potential sources of life, and a few Hindus may be prepared to eat them for this reason. Many vegetarian Hindus however feel as revolted by the idea of eating eggs as they do by the idea of eating meat.

Cheese

Most Asian people who came to Britain as adults do not

eat Western cheese because they find it rancid and very strong. Most Western cheese is anyway, strictly speaking, unsuitable for vegetarians since it is made with animal rennet, though many Hindu vegetarians now accept it. Cottage and curd cheeses and vegetarian cheeses which are not made with animal rennet are completely acceptable in religious terms.

9.2 Other food restrictions

Many of the restrictions connected with the Hindu caste system relate to food. Cooked food is considered to be easily polluted, and, in strict Hindu tradition, cannot be eaten if for example it has been touched by someone of a lower caste. Most Hindus in Britain do not adhere to these very strict prohibitions, but some, generally older people, will eat only food prepared at home by a member of their own family. A very few may even refuse to drink water outside their home and may always carry drinking water with them. Glass and stainless steel are believed to retain pollution less than china or plastic; some people may prefer to drink tea and other drinks out of a glass.

In Asian tradition beliefs about food are part of a whole science based on maintaining a physical and emotional equilibrium. What you eat affects the whole of you: spiritually and emotionally as well as physically. Certain foods, for example onions, garlic and chillies, are believed to raise the body temperature, excite the emotions, and increase activity. These may be known as 'hot foods' (this has nothing to do with temperature). Other foods — 'cold foods' — are believed to cool the body temperature, calm the emotions, and make a person cheerful and strong. Too many of either can unbalance the body and the emotions and cause problems. Maintaining a balance of foods, and ensuring physical and emotional health and equilibrium are considered part of one's religious duty. Beliefs about hot and cold foods are most likely to be followed by older people within the Asian communities, or at important times such as during and after pregnancy and during illness. This may affect the acceptability of dietary advice. It is important to check that people feel able to eat the foods that are advised.

Some conservative Hindus, including members of the Swami Harayan sect, do not eat onions or garlic, which are hot foods and are believed to be harmful stimulants. They may also avoid root vegetables. Some Hindus also avoid tea and coffee as stimulants.

In Hindu tradition, elderly people should withdraw from the rush and concerns of daily life, and should concentrate on spiritual matters. They should eat little, and only foods that are considered pure. Elderly people, particularly widows, may be careful about what they eat, and may also fast several days a week.

9.3 Providing food in hospital

A strict vegetarian Hindu cannot eat meat, fish, eggs or meat products. Anything containing non-vegetarian ingredients is also prohibited: puddings containing suet, cakes cooked in tins greased with lard or containing eggs. Since the name of a dish often gives no clue to its ingredients and since Asian people may not be familiar with British recipes, many people will refuse all but the plainest boiled or fresh vegetables and fruit. If a devout Hindu does not know what is in a dish and what cooking fat was used he or she cannot eat it. People who do not read English will need additional help in choosing acceptable dishes from the menu.

Most vegetarian Hindus will not eat any food that has been in contact with prohibited foods: a salad from which a slice of ham or roast beef has been removed has already been contaminated. Utensils that have not been washed since they last touched prohibited food, contaminate any other food that they touch; the same spoon must not be used to serve potatoes for vegetarian Hindus and stew for other patients. This is really important and most vegetarians will be very concerned about it.

Some conservative Hindus, particularly elderly people, consider that if a utensil has ever been used for a prohibited food it contaminates all other foods. They will refuse all food that has been prepared outside their own homes.

In hospitals and other institutions it may be impossible to keep utensils and cooking pots completely separate. Most devout Hindus feel able to accept this so long as they are sure that all utensils and cooking pots have been well washed since they last touched prohibited food.

In cases where Hindu patients are unable to eat any of the

food offered by the hospital and where no other foods are available, it may be possible to provide simple but nourishing snacks until more suitable food can be found. Salad, milk, fresh or dried fruit, vegetables and nuts will almost always be acceptable.

9.4 Fasting

Some Hindus, especially women, may fast on several days a year: Mahashivratri (in February or March), Ram Naumi (in March or April), Janmastami (in August or September). Some devout Hindus may also make regular fasts, for example on one or two days of special religious significance every week or on two days a month to mark the waxing and waning of the moon. The particular days will depend on which religious sect someone belongs to or which deity they worship (see 4.7 above). Many Hindu women in Britain, for example, fast on Tuesdays. Men may fast on Saturdays. Some Hindus fast on days with a certain astrological significance.

Individuals may also abstain from certain foods for longer continuous periods for a special intention, such as a successful pregnancy or the recovery of a relative. On one particular day every October, Karva Chot, many Hindu women abstain from food from dawn until they see the moon, to ensure that their husbands remain healthy and happy. Unmarried Hindu girls may make a similar fast for their future husbands at Jaya Parvati in July. Some women eat an entirely salt-free diet for one month every year.

A Hindu fast does not necessarily involve abstaining from all food, although some people do make a complete fast. More usually, people who are fasting eat one meal a day, eating only foods that are considered pure, such as fruit or yoghurt, nuts or potatoes, or avoiding salty or less pure foods. They may refuse medication. Details will vary. In Britain, the elderly and women who do not go out to work are most likely to be able to fast regularly.

Fasting is believed to bring both physical and spiritual benefits. Like many Christians, many Hindus believe that they can influence future events by individual acts of devotion, prayer and sacrifice. Fasting is therefore both a means of spiritual purification and can also help to ensure future happiness and security for oneself or one's family. In physical terms fasting is regarded as very important and healthy. It purifies and calms the body and the digestive system.

People in hospital who are not seriously ill may wish to maintain their regular pattern of fasts. Find out whether Hindu patients in hospital wish to fast, what foods they can and cannot eat, and when they wish to eat. Fasting in hospital should not normally present major problems for staff.*

9.5 Alcohol
Alcohol is not permitted as it prevents people from being fully in control of themselves. A few Westernised Hindus may drink but this is generally disapproved of by conservative members of the community.

9.6 Tobacco
Tobacco is generally regarded as a harmful narcotic and most devout Hindus do not smoke.

*For more information about Asian dietary patterns see *Asian Foods & Diets* in this series, available from the National Extension College.

10. Family planning

10.1 Contraception

In the Indian subcontinent attitudes to contraception vary widely and are influenced by many factors including class, economic status, occupation, religion, type of family, and whether people live in urban or rural areas. For most Hindus there seems to be no specific religious ruling either permitting or prohibiting artificial methods of birth control, though members of some sects may follow special rulings. Both religious and cultural traditions, however, stress the value of the family, children as the purpose of marriage, and motherhood as women's chief joy and fulfilment. At the same time there is widespread propaganda in India recommending contraception and smaller families.

In rural Asian societies a large family with several sons ensures family prosperity and survival and is regarded as a blessing. Traditional Hindu couples are likely to continue to feel that a large family is desirable and to see children as the focus of family life. In addition it is most important that a Hindu couple should have at least one son so that he can light the funeral pyre at his father's cremation. It is traditionally believed that a man without a son to perform this crucial rite will suffer in his next life. Many Hindu couples will therefore decide to continue having children until they have at least one son.

Hindu couples from East Africa and younger Hindu couples in Britain are more likely to decide to limit or space their families in line with current British trends.

For some women, certain contraceptive methods may cause particular problems: for example a method that causes spotting or irregular periods, or particularly long periods, may be unattractive to a woman whose religious and household activities are restricted during menstruation. Some women find internal examinations shocking and humiliating they may not wish to use any contraceptive method that requires one. Some people may reject an IUD on the grounds that it is an abortifacient. The decision is a personal one for every woman, and religious and cultural factors are likely to be important in influencing her choice.

10.2 Abortion

Abortion is traditionally disapproved of but individual attitudes may differ a good deal. Many women will only consider abortion if their situation is desperate, for example, if an unmarried woman becomes pregnant.

Younger people may be influenced by current British attitudes and may accept abortion more easily, though it will still be most important to maintain confidentiality.

10.3 Infertility

The overwhelming importance of children, and especially of sons, in Asian culture can have serious implications in cases of infertility or related problems. As used to be the case in Britain, women are generally considered responsible for the ability to produce children, and a wife who cannot have children is likely to feel herself a failure as a woman. Her husband and in-laws may in some cases reject her, and failure to produce a child may lead to divorce. In some families failure to produce sons may also be regarded as cause for rejecting a wife. In a few rare cases the husband may take a second wife, though he must discuss this with his first wife and get permission from her.

Men may be extremely reluctant to attend infertility clinics with their wives and may feel humiliated and angry at any suggestion that they are in some way responsible. Considerable tact and time may be required to overcome this problem.

The procedures of an infertility clinic are anyway likely to be completely unfamiliar and possibly very offensive. Patients whose English is not very good will need an interpreter. The interpreter should be of the same sex as the patient and should be married.

11. The caste system

Hindu society is traditionally divided into many hundreds of interdependent castes, based on social and occupational status and on geographical area of residence. These castes are grouped together into four main varna (social categories).

The origins of the caste system go back many thousands of years. Many Hindus would say that caste divisions originally represented the spiritual levels attained by different groups, and that in the beginning it was possible for people to rise from one caste or subcaste to another as they became spiritually more enlightened.

The exclusive and hierarchical caste structure however became entrenched, and developed into an extremely rigid structure in which each individual's social and spiritual status, occupation, social contacts and social and religious duties were all defined according to the caste and subcaste into which they were born, and could not be changed.

11.1 The theory of the caste system

The different varna with their clearly fixed hereditary duties, rights and relationships were defined with religious force in the Laws of Manu, compiled by Manu, an Indian sage, in about 200 B.C. These describe the symbolic relationship of the four different categories.

The highest category, the Brahmins, symbolised the mouth of Brahman, the Supreme Being. They were the priests within society. Their duty was to study and expound the sacred writings, to conduct religious ceremonies, and to teach the people. Priests in Hindu temples still generally come from the Brahmin caste.

The second category was the Kshatriyas who symbolised the arms of Brahman. Their social duty was to defend and govern the people. In theory they were the politically dominant group.

The third category was the Vaishyas, who symbolised the thighs of Brahman. Their social duty was to produce the food and goods on which all other people depended; they were the farmers, craftsmen and tradesmen.

The fourth category was the Shudras, who symbolised the feet of Brahman. Their social duty was to serve the other three categories.

The symbolic relationship of the four varna indicates their interdependence; a head cannot function without a body; each part needs and is needed by the other three parts. No part can perform the tasks of any other part.

In any Indian village a number of separate groups can be found, each linked by descent to a particular occupation. The Hindi word for these groups is jati; the best English translation is caste. Each caste is a local group and will have members in several local villages. People marry within their own caste, but outside their own village. In traditional village society each caste only performs a certain task, e.g. farming, making pots, weaving, performing religious ceremonies, and relies on members of other castes in the village to provide the things or perform the tasks that it cannot.

In some ways the Hindu caste system can be likened historically to a system of exclusive trades unions in which the members of each union can only perform their own set of tasks, but in which by all working together the members combine to achieve their overall goal. To take one example, in an Indian village the Brahmins are traditionally called on by other families to perform religious ceremonies, bless special events, read horoscopes and so forth. In return those families who farm provide them with food, those families who make pots or do carpentry provide them with what they produce, and so on. However, with increasing mobility, industrialisation and outside influence this strong system of mutual dependence is beginning to break down, especially in urban areas, though it is still an ideal of co-operation to which many Hindus hold.

According to Manu, the higher the caste to which anyone belonged, the greater were their spiritual duties and responsibilities and the more strictly they had to observe rules concerning diet, worship, social contact, avoidance of pollution and so on. This still holds true to a large extent. Traditional Brahmins, for example, are more likely to be careful about following a vegetarian diet and not drinking alcohol, about ensuring that all utensils are clean, about showering frequently and changing their clothes, about praying and worshipping regularly, and about bringing up their children in the same way. People from other caste groups are not expected to follow as strict a routine. Each group has different duties and obligations to fulfil.

The caste into which each individual was born is determined by their karma, the cycle of reward and punishment. The caste system is therefore strongly tied in with reincarnation and so has religious force. It is regarded by many Hindus as divinely ordained and part of natural law.

In traditional Indian society, as well as the members of the castes corresponding to the four main social categories, there are people who exist on the fringes of society and belong to no caste. They do the jobs that are considered spiritually polluting, such as cleaning streets and lavatories. They used to be known as Outcastes or Untouchables. Strictly speaking they have no social relationship with anyone within the caste system. They live apart from other people and do not mix with them.

Mahatma Gandhi (1869–1948), who like many earlier Hindu reformers fought against the caste system, was particularly concerned to raise the status of the Outcastes. He called them Harijans, Children of God, and made a point of mixing and eating with them. It is now illegal in India to discriminate on grounds of caste, and a special number of places are reserved in colleges, universities and in the civil service for Harijans, or Scheduled Castes as they are now officially known.

The caste system has existed for thousands of years, during which different caste groups have lived completely separately, mixing little except in defined functional roles, and intermarrying rarely. The caste system has religious backing and so is seen by many devout Hindus as a proper division of society. Despite the pressures of the twentieth century therefore, it is slow to change, and caste identity and feeling are likely to remain even among people who no longer follow the traditional occupation of their caste.

11.2 Belonging to a caste

Each caste contains several thousand people and originates from a specific geographical area. All the members of each caste traditionally follow the same occupation, and worship in the same way. They often share the same family names. It is normal for people to marry within their own caste.

In many ways the people of each caste see themselves as the members of one community, more or less as cousins, with strong mutual responsibilities and a sense of close relationship and warmth. Most people marry and mix socially within their own caste group. One's relations and friends are therefore often members of one's own caste. The family, and its extension the caste, are the two most important units to which each person belongs. People may look to other members of their caste for support and company and for financial help, for example, for a loan for a house, or for money for a good cause.

11.3 Caste in Britain

In Britain caste awareness is likely to remain strong, like class awareness among older and more traditional people, particularly among those who came to Britain as adults. Caste bonds were also very important to new arrivals in the first years of migration and settlement, and several caste-based welfare organisations developed for the support of members in need. Most Hindu organisations are still organised within caste groupings. However, since Hindus in Britain no longer follow traditional caste-based occupations, and since traditional differences in wealth between the castes are not maintained here, differences are becoming increasingly blurred. They are unlikely to affect people outside the Hindu communities.

Caste is however still likely to be very important when it comes to marriage; most Hindu parents will disapprove strongly of anyone marrying outside their caste, and may refuse to allow such a marriage. They are likely to believe that for social, religious and economic reasons, their children should marry within their own caste. Caste may also affect how people feel about their place in society.

12. Hindu names

Hindu names from northern India generally work on a system similar to the British naming system. However, forms of address are different and this can lead to confusion when addressing patients or clients or recording their names.

The system described here refers mainly to the names of Hindus whose families originated in Punjab and Gujarat. The naming system of Hindus from other parts of India may differ to some extent.

Hindus in Britain from East Africa are used to many of the features of life in a Western-influenced bureaucracy. They are likely to give their names in a way that fits into British records, and there is less likely to be confusion with their names in records.

12.1 The Hindu naming system

The basic Hindu naming system has three parts, much like the British naming system.

Lalitadevi	Patel	(f)
Rajkumar	Sharma	(m)
Vijaykumar	Patel	(m)

The first part: Lalita, Raj, Vijay, is the *personal name,* as in the British system, and is the name used by family and close friends.

The second part: Devi, Kumar, the *middle name*, is only used with the first name. It cannot be used as a separate name on its own. The first and middle names are often used together to address an older person or to show respect. This (i.e. not title + surname as in the British system) is the traditional Hindu polite form of address.

There are a number of common Hindu middle names which it is easy to recognise:

Female: Behn, Devi, Gowri, Kumari, Lakshmi, Rani

Male: Bhai, Chand, Das, Dev, Kant, Kumar, Lal, Nath, Pal

In Indian languages when both first and middle names are used they are always written together: Lalitadevi, Vijaykumar. In British records they may be written separately: Lalita Devi, Vijay Kumar.

The third part: Sharma, Patel, is the *surname*, the family name. The family name is often a caste name, shared by some or all of the members of one caste. Because most Hindus in Britain come from only a few castes, and from two main geographical areas (Gujarat and Punjab) many Hindu families in Britain share the same caste or family name, and certain names, such as Patel (a Gujarati caste name) are very common.

As in the British system, wives and children take their husband's or father's surname.

In Britain, some Hindu parents give their children only a first name and a surname, omitting the traditional middle name: Lalita Patel, Raj Sharma.

12.2 Common mistakes with Hindu names in records

Duplicate records

Because the traditional polite or formal Hindu form of address is to give first name and middle name only, with no surname, Hindu names have often been entered wrongly in British records.

For example: Lakshmidevi Vasani gave her name as Lakshmidevi when she first arrived in Britain. This is the way in which she would normally give it in India and within her own community. A British receptionist, used to and expecting first name and surname, wrote down Devi as the surname and Lakshmi as the first name. Lakshmidevi was then addressed and recorded incorrectly, as Mrs Devi. Her husband and children were wrongly assumed also to have the surname Devi. When Lakshmidevi realised that in Britain the family name is used in formal situations she started to give her full name: Lakshmidevi Vasani. She now has duplicate records;

one (incorrectly) under Devi, and a second (correctly) under Vasani.

A Hindu middle name entered as a surname in records is almost always wrong (see 12.3 below for a very rare exception). Ask for the family name. Enter this as a surname. Make sure that all records are now filed under that name.

Common surnames

In areas where a large Hindu community from one region has settled, many families have the same surname. Enter each person's father's or husband's name as well to help with the identification of records. This is the established Hindu system (see 12.3).

12.3 Possible variations in Hindu names

Dropping the surname

A very few Hindus have dropped their family name to indicate rejection of the caste system. (This is very rare with Gujarati Hindus, the majority in Britain). They will use their middle name, e.g. Devi, Nath, as a surname. Each member of a family will then usually have a different surname, for example, Mr Nath will be married to Mrs Devi. Or occasionally, the whole family will adopt what is in fact the father's middle name e.g. Nath, as their surname.

Note that this variation is rare. In almost all cases, if a Hindu middle name is down in records as a surname this is a mistake: correct it as described in 12.2 above.

Gujarati Hindu names

Among Gujarati Hindus it is traditional for men and single women to use their father's name and for married women to use their husband's name after their own first and middle name.

For example: Vijaykumar is the son of Jayantilal Patel. He usually gives his name as Vijaykumar Jayantilal Patel.

Vijaykumar's wife is called Lakshmidevi. She usually gives her name as Lakshmidevi Vijaykumar Patel. Their son Subashbhai usually gives his name as Subashbhai Vijaykumar Patel. Their daughter Neeshagowri, gives her name as Neeshagowri Vijaykumar Patel until she marries. When she marries she replaces her father's name with her husband's.

This system helps to distinguish people with common family names. Many Hindus in Britain still use it, but some drop their father's or husband's name when dealing with British officials, shortening the name for the purpose of British records, and so losing an important item of extra identification.

12.4 Forms of address

Formal usage

The traditional Hindu polite form of address is first name + middle name:

Lalitadevi

Vijaykumar

Sometimes, particularly among Hindus, the first name + bhai, meaning brother, or behn, meaning sister, is used as the polite form of address:

Lalitabehn

Vijaybhai or Vijaykumarbhai

This is more or less equivalent to the British polite form of title + surname.

In Britain it is usually acceptable to use title and family name:

Mrs Sharma

Mr Patel

It is also acceptable to use title + full name:

Mrs Lalitadevi Sharma

Mr Vijaykumar Patel

The Indian equivalent of Mr and Mrs are Shri and Shrimati:

Shrimati Lalitadevi Sharma

Shri Vijaykumar Patel

Shri may also be used to show respect:

Shri Bhagavad Gita (the holy book)

Shri Krishna (an incarnation of Vishnu)

The suffix —ji may also be added to a name to show respect and affection:

Gandhiji

Krishnaji

Informal usage

For children or for close friends use the first name alone, as in Britain:

Lalita
Vijay*

---

*For more details on the Hindu and other Asian naming systems and specific guidance on how to record and use them, see *Asian Names and Records* in this series, available from the National Extension College, 18 Brooklands Avenue, Cambridge CB2 2HN.

13. Birth and childhood ceremonies

Customs connected with birth and childhood vary a good deal between communities and between families. Some of the more common are outlined here. The extent to which traditional customs and ceremonies are retained or modified by families living in Britain will also vary.

13.1 At the birth

As soon as possible after a Hindu baby is born a member of the family may write 'OM', a mystical sound representing the Supreme Spirit, on the baby's tongue with honey or with ghee. The man or woman who does this will take on a role similar to that of a Christian godparent towards the child. In Britain this ceremony may be delayed until the mother and baby have returned home from hospital.

Most Hindu parents will wish to have their child's horoscope read by an astrologer, often a priest. Astrological influences are generally believed to have a strong influence on each individual's character, personality and future. In the same way as all life and all living things are interdependent, so human beings are influenced by inanimate objects outside themselves and by the movement of the stars and planets.

It will be important for many Hindu parents to know the exact time of their child's birth in order to get an accurate horoscope made out. Horoscopes are likely to be consulted, for example, before a marriage is arranged, to ensure that the couple are compatible. Certain days and times are also considered particularly auspicious and suitable for a wedding, a special event, a ceremony, an operation or a journey.

On the sixth day after a birth the women of the family may gather to give thanks, to congratulate the mother and to bring presents for her and the child. Women in Britain may come to visit a new mother who is still in hospital for this special celebration.

The sixth day is also the day on which Hindus traditionally believe that a child's fate is written. Some parents may leave a symbolic blank sheet of paper and a pen near the baby's cot. They may make an offering to Saraswati, goddess of learning.

13.2 Naming the child

Children are traditionally given their chosen name by a priest at the mandir (temple) on the tenth day after the birth but this may be delayed in Britain.

The first letter of a baby's name is often decided by the astrologer, usually a priest, who makes out the baby's horoscope. An older member of the family, a grandparent or an older aunt, then usually chooses a name beginning with that letter. If the relative choosing the name is in India or East Africa it may take some time for the final decision to get back to Britain. In such cases a family may use and even register the child under a nickname or temporary name until the final name arrives. Nicknames for children are anyway very common, especially if the chosen name is something of a mouthful.

13.3 Childhood ceremonies

In some families the head of a small boy, and occasionally of a girl, is shaved by a priest at a family celebration. One small lock of hair is usually left on the head. This may be done about six weeks after the birth, or later. It is sometimes done when a boy is a year old. It may also be delayed until the child is on a visit to India and makes a pilgrimage to a special shrine.

In some Hindu families of higher castes, when a boy reaches the age of seven, the age at which he begins to reason and to be able to distinguish right and wrong, a sacred thread is put around his body and over one shoulder to mark the beginning of his religious awareness and adult status. Very few Hindu families follow this custom in Britain (see also 8.2 above).

14. Marriage

For Hindus, as for Christians, marriage is a sacrament as well as a contract and a social ceremony. The sacrament of marriage is very highly valued. It is considered that every Hindu should marry and raise a family and that marriage is the beginning of a more responsible and purposeful life.

In Asian tradition marriages are usually arranged by the families of the young people concerned, though this practice is changing in the subcontinent and in East Africa as well as in Britain. Young people nowadays generally play an important part in choosing their partner. Nevertheless, marriage is still seen very much as a union between and a matter for two whole families, not just as a private union between two individuals.

Hindu marriages are almost always arranged within the same caste and the couple's horoscopes are consulted to ensure that they will be compatible. Some Hindu communities give large dowries with their daughters. In such communities to give one's daughter a good dowry becomes very important, and this can lead to real hardship for families with several daughters. In some Gujarati communities in Britain, a dowry is given with the son.

Traditionally wedding ceremonies and celebrations last several days and often take place in the open air. In Britain however, because of the climate and the press of daily life, a wedding usually only lasts one day, takes place on a Saturday or Sunday, and is usually held in a hall. As many friends and relatives as possible are invited and the women of the families spend weeks beforehand preparing food, making clothes and so forth. As in British and most Asian traditions, the bride's family usually pays for the wedding and is responsible for all the food and hospitality.

Both the bride and the groom go through various ceremonies before the wedding itself. The wedding ceremony, with a priest officiating, usually takes place in front of a large group of assembled friends and relatives. During the short ceremony the bride and groom receive symbolic gifts to bring them good fortune, prosperity, and a happy stable marriage. The bride and groom walk several times round a small fire, which symbolises purity, while the congregation sings. They promise to stay together as long as they live, to take each other as their beloved, to care for each other, and to share each other's problems. Then guests give the couple presents, congratulate them and wish them well. They may sprinkle rice on the couple to symbolise happiness and wealth. Presents are also given by each family to the other. After the ceremony there is usually a wedding reception.

Widowhood

Hinduism stresses the sanctity of marriage and particularly its importance for women. Traditionally a woman whose husband dies should withdraw from social and family life and should lead a sober and quiet life remaining spiritually bound to her husband. Because of karma, the system of reward and punishment for previous deeds, a widow may be seen as in some way responsible for her widowhood.

When her husband dies a widow removes and breaks her wedding bangles and any other wedding jewellery. Many widows, particularly older women, wear only white to indicate their withdrawal from the world. Widows do not wear a bindi or dye the partings of their hair. Traditionally a Hindu widow could never remarry and had to remain dependent on her husband's or her own family. Nowadays, however, attitudes are changing and young widows are likely to remarry. The stigma attached to widows is beginning to die out, and there are few restrictions on their behaviour.

Divorce

Marriage is regarded by Hindus as a holy and indissoluble sacrament. Divorce goes very much against this tradition. Although divorce has been permitted for Hindus under Indian law since 1955, it is extremely rare in conservative communities. In Britain the divorce rate among Hindus is increasing, but divorce is still regarded by most people as shameful, and only occurs when the marital situation is desperate.

There is a strong stigma against divorced people, particularly women. A woman who seeks a divorce may be risking social disapproval and rejection by her community. However, a younger divorced woman may marry again.

15. Death and cremation

15.1 Care of the dying

A devout Hindu who is very ill or dying may receive comfort from hymns and readings from the Hindu holy books, especially the Bhagavad Gita.

Some families may wish to call a Hindu priest to perform holy rites. He may tie a thread around the neck or wrist of the dying person to bless them. This should not be removed. The priest may also sprinkle blessed water from the Ganges over the dying person or place a sacred tulsi leaf or blessed water in his or her mouth.

If no family member is present it is probably best for hospital staff to contact the local Hindu temple, provided the patient wishes, to ask someone to come and attend the patient. The hospital chaplain may also be able to give help and advice.

A dying Hindu patient may wish very much to die at home. This has religious significance, and great distress may be caused to the dying person and to the family if he or she dies in hospital. Provided the family wishes, all possible steps should be taken to enable the patient to go home to die.

Some devout Hindus, when they are dying, may wish to lie on the floor, symbolising closeness to Mother Earth.

15.2 Last offices

A few families are very particular about who touches a dead relative's body. For a non-Hindu to touch or wash the body may sometimes cause real distress. It is important to ask the family about this as about all other procedures. If no friend or relative is available, guidance should be sought from the local Hindu temple.

Unless the family instructs otherwise, the following should be done: Close the eyes and straighten the limbs. If the body must not be touched health workers should use disposable gloves. Jewellery, sacred threads and other religious objects should not be removed. The body should be wrapped in a plain sheet without a religious emblem. In most cases it should not be washed: this is part of the funeral rites and will usually be carried out by relatives later.

The body is then usually taken home and washed and laid out. The eldest son is usually in charge of funeral arrangements. The body is wrapped in a white cotton shroud or white clothes. A young bride may be wrapped in a red cotton shroud.

A coin, a small piece of gold or a leaf from the sacred tulsi plant may be placed in the dead person's mouth. Some Hindu families in Britain may ask for the body to be taken to an undertaker's rather than to their house.

15.3 Post-mortems etc.

There is no specific religious prohibition against post-mortem examinations but many people may find them aborrent. It is important that cremation should take place as soon as possible. There is no prohibition against blood transfusions, organ transplants or any other medical procedure.

15.4 Cremation

All adult Hindus are cremated. Young children and infants are usually buried. Cremation or burial should take place as soon as possible, and in India it is usually done within twenty-four hours. Families may keep an oil lamp burning in the room with the dead person until the cremation takes place.

There may be a special service before the cremation. This service is usually held at home but in Britain it may be held at a Chapel of Rest. Several important ceremonies take place before the cremation. These may include placing religious and other objects beside the body in the coffin.

Traditionally the eldest son has the sacred duty of igniting the funeral pyre. He will probably expect to press the button at the crematorium and this can usually be arranged.

During the cremation prayers are chanted and hymns read.

Afterwards the ashes are collected and are often taken back to India to be scattered in a sacred river, particularly the River Ganga, the most sacred river of Hinduism. If this is not possible they may be scattered in a British river or in the sea.

The family and relatives return home in mourning after the cremation. Most people will take a full shower when they get home to wash away the spiritual pollution of death.

In the days following the death the whole family is in mourning. Relatives and close friends will come to keep the family company and comfort them, and to share their grief and support them. Members of the close family, particularly women, may sometimes not eat until the cremation has taken place. This is one reason why it should take place as soon as possible. Older women may mourn in the traditional manner, wailing and keening loudly to show their grief. The family may wear white, usually for the first ten days after the death, as a sign of mourning. The widow and eldest son of a dead man may shave their heads. Members of the family say special prayers and eat only simple food. They may hold a reading of one of the holy books.

Coping with the unfamiliar organisational side of death and cremation in Britain can be extremely distressing for bereaved relatives. Practical help is often needed, for example in contacting undertakers and explaining what is required, contacting employers, dealing with paperwork and so forth.

15.5 Anniversaries

On the anniversary of the death of a parent, grandparent, or great grandparent, families may hold a special ceremony of worship and prayer for their souls. It is important to have children to ensure this benefit for oneself and one's parents and grandparents.

16. Different Hindu communities in Britain

Since Hindu beliefs and practices are not centrally regulated or co-ordinated, people from each different area, caste and sect will tend to form a cohesive community that worships and socialises together. Each community will adhere to different practices and different details of belief and will usually have its own local temple. Members of the same community settled in different areas of Britain often visit each other for special social and religious events and usually maintain close links, much like a very large family.

Each Hindu community will differ: members of some are particularly strict about adhering to dietary restrictions and avoiding any food prepared outside the home; some sects follow a living spiritual leader; some are highly organised with a formal centralised structure, welfare provision and fund-raising procedures; some are exclusive, and some are merely loose groups of people from the same area with similar beliefs; in some communities or sects the members follow a strict code of discipline, in others they do not. Except among the most exclusive sects there is no hostility or sense of superiority towards Hindus who follow other practices and beliefs. Depending on the main manifestation of the Supreme Spirit worshipped by its members, each community will celebrate certain special festivals.

From the point of view of health workers the community or sect to which an individual or a family belongs is particularly likely to be significant in two main respects: firstly with regard to diet, religious ceremonies and formal prayer in hospitals, though even within each Hindu community individual practices vary a good deal; and secondly with regard to who, within the local Hindu communities, can be called on for advice and support when necessary. Like Christians, Hindus will generally feel most at ease with members of their own sect or community.

17. Hindu festivals

The two most important Hindu festivals are Holi and Diwali. These are celebrated by all Hindus.

In India Holi and Diwali are celebrated with holidays and family celebrations in the same way as Christmas in Britain. Most Hindu patients in hospital would like to go home over these two holidays if possible, in the same way as many patients are allowed home over Christmas. Non-urgent tests, operations, or investigations for Hindus should be avoided as far as possible over these festivals. Routine home visits should wait where possible till afterwards. It is important to know the dates of Holi and Diwali each year in order to plan around them with patients and their families.

Hindu patients in hospital over Holi or Diwali are likely to receive cards and presents very much as at Christmas. Family and friends may wish to visit throughout the day, bringing special festive sweets and other dishes. Patients who are on a restricted diet should be allowed a taste of these if at all possible. Relatives may also bring sweets or cakes to share with the other patients on the ward.

Hindu patients may like to get together during Holi and Diwali in much the same way as would English people in hospital abroad over Christmas and will be grateful for recognition that this is a special festive time for them. It may be possible to discuss in advance the significance of Holi and Diwali and what provision Hindu patients would like. Staff and other patients should be encouraged to wish any Hindu patients Happy Holi or Happy Diwali.

The Hindu Year

The dates of most Hindu festivals vary slightly from year to year, depending on the moon.

October/ November	*Bestuvarash: New Year's Day* The day after Diwali, the beginning of the Hindu year.
February/ March	*Mahashivratri* Birth of Shiva. Some people fast until about 4 o'clock in the afternoon when a ceremony is held at the temple. Celebrations at night, feasting the next day.
February/ March (full moon)	*Holi* Hindu Spring Festival celebrated in northern and central India. Celebrates an ancient legend in which Good triumphs over Evil, now often associated with Krishna. A bonfire is lit and ceremonies held at the temple. In India celebrations and festivities last three days.
March/April	*Ram Naumi* Birth of Rama, incarnation of Vishnu, and hero of the epic poem the Ramayana. Many people fast during the day, avoiding, for example, vegetables, cereals and salt. Celebrations at night.
August (full moon)	*Raksha Bandhan* Celebration of the bond between brothers and sisters. Sisters make or buy string or tinsel bracelets (rakhi) which they tie on their brother's wrists. Brothers give gifts in return and promise to support and protect their sisters all their lives.
August/ September	*Janmastami* Birth of Krishna. Celebrated mainly in northern and central India. Some people fast all day the day before until the celebration of the birth at midnight. Many people spend the whole night celebrating and singing in the temple. People may fast on the following day.
August/ September	*Ganesh Chaturthi* Festival of Ganesh, the god of Prosperity and Good Fortune, son of Shiva and Parvati. Celebrated especially in central and western India.

September/ October	*Navratri* Festival of nine nights leading up to Dussehra. Festival of young girls and women who dress up and sing and dance and celebrate for nine evenings. Some people may fast for the nine days eating only sweet milky dishes and fruit. Dedicated to the mother goddess Durga or Amba.
October	*Dussehra* (known as *Durga Puja* in Bengal) Tenth day, at the end of Navratri celebration of the mother goddess Durga, the female principle of Energy and Motherhood. Presents exchanged and family celebration.
October	*Saraswati puja* Celebration of Saraswati, goddess of learning and art.
October/ November	*Diwali* Five-day festival of light and of the goddess Lakshmi, the goddess of Good Fortune and Prosperity. Celebrates the victory of Good over Evil. Candles and lamps are lit in all the houses to celebrate and to guide Lakshmi to the house. Family celebration and present giving, similar to Christmas. Some families may send Diwali cards.

The precise dates of Hindu festivals can usually be obtained each year from your local Community Relations Council or from the Commission for Racial Equality, Elliot House, 10–12 Allington Street, London SW1 5EH (01–828–7022)

18. Note to trainers

This book is not necessarily intended as the basis of a training session, though it can be used as such by people who wish to run a session specifically on aspects of Hinduism and on caring for Hindu patients. It may also be read purely as a source of background information which can then be fed with other information into more general training sessions for health workers and other groups.

18.1 Running a training session on the care of Hindu patients

Religious practices and prohibitions make little sense out of context. The religious practices of non-Christian patients are too often seen merely as difficulties, problems, and sources of inconvenience for health workers — not the ideal starting point for a supportive relationship or for mutual respect. For many Hindu people their religion is the focus of their lives. Consequently, some introduction to the basic ideas behind Hinduism and Hindu practices is essential if health workers are to be equipped to work sensitively and knowledgeably with their Hindu patients and clients.

The type and length of training session to be run will depend on the time available, the amount of knowledge the trainees already have, and whether there is a significant Hindu population living locally. Most non-Hindu trainers and tutors will also be naturally and justifiably reluctant to conduct a training session about a religion of which they are not followers. For this reason Hindu outside speakers who can speak of their own faith and practices and from their own experience, should be brought in wherever possible.

18.2 Suggested aims and content of a training session

Aims

i)   to give trainees a basic understanding of and respect for the fundamental ideas and values of Hinduism

ii) to discuss how far these ideas and values are likely to be important to Hindus in Britain

iii) to describe Hindu religious practices likely to be important to trainees in their work with patients and clients, and to discuss their practical implications

iv) to enable trainees to discuss Hindu beliefs and practices sensitively with Hindu people from a basis of some knowledge and confidence

Content

(Precise content will depend on the needs and situations of trainees.)

1.   The areas of origin of the families of Hindus in Britain

2.   Brief historical outline: development of Hinduism, diversity and underlying uniformity

3.   The main features of the Hindu world-view: the Supreme Spirit, Ultimate Reality; the soul in all living things; respect for life; sansar, the cycle of birth and rebirth; karma, the natural law of reward for past deeds and thoughts; moksha, the goal of release from earthly existence; dharma, right and fitting conduct; the scale of purity and impurity; the Hindu deities

4.   Family and community values: men and women, the elderly, marriage and divorce, family planning; worship at home and at the temple, the role of the temple in the community; the caste system and its importance in Britain

5.   Hospital care: standards of modesty and personal cleanliness, provision in hospital; items of jewellery and makeup, religious and personal significance, implications in hospital; possible dietary restrictions, food in hospital and during illness, appropriate provision, giving dietary advice

6.   The northern Hindu naming system: differences from

the British system, avoiding confusion, pronouncing names correctly

7.   Birth and childhood ceremonies: provision in hospital

8.   Care of the dying: family involvement, last offices, guidance for hospital staff

9.   The major Hindu festivals and their significance: Hindu patients in hospital

10.   The local Hindu community: local temples and other Hindu organisations

18.3 Using outside speakers

Speakers should be asked to spend a good proportion of the session on topics connected with health care and on practices that are likely to be important in caring for people in institutions.

It is important to discuss the aims of the session with them beforehand, as well as any questions or problems that trainees are likely to raise during the session.

It may also be useful to ask the speaker to read quickly through this book to get some idea of the issues that are likely to be important, and to raise and discuss issues on which he or she disagrees. A speaker should bear in mind the regional and class differences that exist between Hindus living in Britain and the need to outline possible variations in practice among local communities.

Local Community Relations Councils, community organisations, colleges or Industrial Language Training Units may be able to suggest suitable speakers. Hindu nurses, doctors or other staff might also be available to speak. In addition, use any Hindu trainees in the group who are prepared to be speakers or additional contributors.

Where it is not possible to get a Hindu speaker to come and talk to trainees, it may at least be possible for the trainer or tutor to visit Hindu patients and families before the session and talk to them about their religious beliefs and practices, the effect of living in Britain on their way of life, the difficulties they face in contacts with the Health Service, what they would like health workers to know about their religion, and how they would like Health Service provision to take account of their religious needs and practices.

APPENDIX: Glossary of Hindu terms and approximate guide to pronunciation

Key to pronunciation

The pronunciation of some words is difficult to indicate in English spelling, but the spellings below give a very rough guide. Pronunciation varies to some extent from area to area. The stressed syllable in each word is italicised, as in *Eng*land and exp*ect*.

Vowels

'*ă*' very short — as in 'material'
'a' short — as in 'must' and 'funny'
'aa' long — as in 'mast' and 'farm'
'o' a rounded 'o' between 'pot' and 'port'
'u' short — as in 'put' and 'foot'
'oo' long — as in 'pool' and 'flu'
'e' short — as in 'pen' and 'fetch'
'i' short — as in 'skip' or 'fist'
'ee' long — as in 'beat' and 'weep'
'ai' — as in 'fight', 'right' and 'kite'
'ay' — as in 'pain' and 'rain'
'au' — as in 'found' and 'round'

Consonants

'r' — is usually pronounced quite strongly
'dh' — is pronounced like 'd' followed by 'h' — as in 'hardhat'
'th' — is not pronounced as it is in English. It is a hard 't' followed by 'h' — as in 'hothouse'
'ss' or 's' — as in 'miss' and 'soon'

Aspirated consonants are not generally indicated.

Achkan (man's long jacket)	*a*chkan
Ahimsa (non-violence)	ah*i*nsaa
Amba (goddess)	amb*aa*
Atman (soul, life force)	*aa*tman
Avatar (incarnation)	av*taa*r
Behn (sister)	bayn
Benares (sacred city)	ban*aa*ress
Bengal (area now divided between India & Bangladesh)	beng*a*wl or b*à*ng*aa*l
Bengali (language or person from West Bengal in India or from Bangladesh)	beng*aa*li
Bhagavad Gita (most popular Hindu Holy Book)	bh*a*gvad g*ee*ta
Bhagwan (Supreme Spirit)	bhagw*aa*n
Bhai (brother)	bhai
Bhai doot (religious spot on man's forehead)	bhai doot
Bhajan (hymn)	bh*a*jan
Bindi (decorative spot on woman's forehead)	b*i*ndi
Brahma (god)	br*a*hmaa
Brahman (Supreme Spirit)	br*aa*hman
Brahmin (member of priestly caste)	br*a*hmin
Buddha (founder of Buddhist religion)	b*u*ddha
Chandlo (Gujarati: decorative spot on woman's forehead)	chandlo
Chuni (long scarf)	chooni
Delhi (capital of India)	d*e*li
Devi (goddess)	d*ay*vi
Dharma (duty, right conduct)	dh*a*rma
Dhoti (male garment)	dh*o*ti
Diwali (festival)	diw*a*li
Dupatta (long scarf)	dup*a*tta
Durga (goddess)	d*u*rga
Durga puja (festival of goddess Durga)	d*u*rga p*oo*ja
Dussehra (festival)	d*à*ss*e*hra
Ganesh (god)	g*à*nesh
Ganesh Chathurthi (festival of Ganesh)	g*à*nesh chat*u*rti
Ganga (sacred river — Ganges)	g*a*nga
Garuda (sun-eagle)	gar*u*d
Ghee (clarified butter)	ghee

Gita (familiar name for Bhagavad Gita)	*gee*ta
Gujarat (Indian State)	gujar*aat*
Gujarati (language or person from Gujarat)	gujar*aati*
Gurdwara (Sikh temple)	g*u*rdwara
Guru (teacher)	g*u*ru
Hanuman (god)	h*a*numan
Harijan (child of god — outcaste)	h*a*rijan
Hawan (fire ceremony)	h*a*wan
Hindi (northern Indian language)	h*i*ndi
Hindu (follower of Hinduism)	h*i*ndu
Holi (festival)	h*o*li
Ishwar (Supreme Spirit)	*ee*shvar
Islam (Muslim religion)	issl*aa*m
Jain (follower of reformist Hindu sect)	jain
Janeu (sacred thread)	jan*ey*oo
Janmastami (festival)	janm*a*shtami
Jati (caste)	j*a*ti
Jaya Parvati (festival)	j*a*ia p*a*rvati
—ji (polite suffix)	—ji
Kameez (shirt)	k*å*m*ee*z
Karma (reward & punishment for past actions)	k*a*rma
Karva Chot (festival)	k*a*rva chot
Kerala (Indian State)	k*e*rala
Krishna (god)	kr*i*shna
Kshatriya (caste)	ksh*a*triya
Kurta (shirt)	k*u*rta
Kutch (northern region of Gujarat)	katch
Kutchi (dialect or person from Kutch)	k*a*tchi
Lakshmi (goddess)	l*a*kshmi
Lingam (phallic emblem)	l*i*ngam
Manabharata (Hindu epic)	mah*aa*bh*aa*rata
Mahadev (name for Shiva)	mah*a*dev
Mahashivratri (festival)	mah*aa*shiv*ra*tri
Mahatma Gandhi (literally Great Soul Gandhi, Indian national hero & leader)	mah*a*tma g*aa*ndhi
Mala (string of prayer beads)	m*aa*la
Malayali (language of Kerala State)	malay*aa*li
Mandir (Hindu temple)	m*a*ndir

Mangal sutra (wedding brooch)	mangàl sutàr
Mantra (prayer)	mantra
Manu (ancient Hindu sage)	manoo
Mataji (mother goddess)	maataji
Moksha (release from cycle of death & rebirth)	moksh
Muslim (follower of Islam)	musslim
Murti (statue)	murti
Nandi (Shiva's bull)	nandi
Navratri (festival)	navratri
Om (sound symbolising Supreme Spirit)	om
Pajama (male garment)	paijama
Pandit (priest)	pandit
Paramatma (Supreme Spirit)	paràmatma
Parameshwar (Supreme Spirit)	parameshwar
Parvati (goddess)	paarvati
Prakash (Supreme Spirit)	prakaash
Puja (worship)	pooja
Punjab (Indian State)	pànjaab
Punjabi (language or person from Punjab)	pànjaabi
Radha (goddess)	raadha
Rakhi (string of tinsel bracelet)	rakhi
Raksha bandhan (festival)	raksha bandhan
Ram Naumi (festival)	raam naumi
Rama (god)	raama
Ramayana (epic poem)	raamaayan
Ravana (demon king in Ramayana)	raavan
Sansar (cycle of birth & rebirth)	sansaar
Sanskrit (ancient language)	sanskrit
Saraswati (goddess)	saraswati
Saraswati puja (festival)	saraswati pooja
Sari (female garment)	saari
Shakh (energy)	shakti
Shalwar (female garment)	shalwaar
Shankar (name of Shiva)	shankar
Shiva (god)	shiva
Shri (Hindi equivalent of Mr.)	shree
Shrimati (Hindi equivalent of Mrs.)	sheemati
Shudra (caste)	shoodra
Sikh (follower of the Sikh religion)	sik or seek

Sindur (red in parting of a woman's hair)	sind*oo*r
Sita (goddess)	s*ee*ta
Swami (teacher)	sw*a*mi
Swami Narayan (founder of a Hindu sect, also name of the sect or follower)	sw*a*mi n*aa*rayan
Tamil (language or person from Tamilnadu State)	t*a*mil
Tamilnadu (Indian State)	t*a*miln*a*d
Tika (religious spot on man's forehead)	t*ee*ka
Tilak (religious spot on woman's forehead)	t*i*lak
Upanishads (sacred texts)	*u*panishads
Vaishnav (worshipper of Vishnu)	v*a*ishnav
Vaishya (caste)	v*a*ishya
Varanasi (sacred city on River Ganga — Benares)	Var*aa*nassi
Varna (caste)	v*a*rna
Veda (revealed scriptures)	v*e*da
Vishnu (god)	v*i*shnu

Bibliography and sources

Bibliographical and sources

Bowen, David G. (ed.), *Hinduism in England*, Faculty of Contemporary Studies, Bradford College 1981

Bridger, Peter, *A Hindu Family in Britain*, Religious Education Press 1977

Crompton, Yorke, *Hinduism*, Ward Lock 1971

Ewan, John, *Understanding Your Hindu Neighbour*, Lutterworth 1977

Harrison, Stephen W., *Hinduism in Preston*, 1978

Iqbal, Muhammed et al., *East Meets West*, Commission for Racial Equality 1981

Mascaro, Juan (trans.), *The Upanishads*, Penguin 1970

Mascaro, Juan (trans.), *The Bhagavad Gita*, Penguin 1975

Narayan, R.K., *Gods, Demons & Others*, Heinemann 1965

Narayan, R.K., *Mahabharata*, Heinemann 1978

Radhakrishnan, *The Hindu View of Life*, Unwin 1971

Thomas, P., *Epics, Myths & Legends of India*, Taraporevala, Bombay 1973

Yogeshananda, Swami, *The Way of the Hindu*, Hulton 1977

For more general information about the health care of Asian people see Henley, Alix, *Asian Patients in Hospital and at Home*, published by King's Fund/Pitman Medical 1979.